T5-BCK-335

The Pharmacy Technician's

Pocket Drug Reference

2ND EDITION

JOYCE A. GENERALI, MS, RPh, FASHP
DIRECTOR, DRUG INFORMATION CENTER
UNIVERSITY OF KANSAS MEDICAL CENTER
KANSAS CITY, KANSAS
CLINICAL ASSOCIATE PROFESSOR
UNIVERSITY OF KANSAS SCHOOL OF PHARMACY
LAWRENCE, KANSAS

APhA

AMERICAN PHARMACEUTICAL ASSOCIATION
WASHINGTON, D.C.

EDITOR: JULIAN I. GRAUBART
LAYOUT AND GRAPHICS: TAMRA ROBERTS

© 2003 by the American Pharmaceutical Association
Published by the American Pharmaceutical
Association, 2215 Constitution Avenue, N.W.,
Washington, DC 20037-2985 (http://www.aphanet.org
Printed in Canada

To comment on this book via e-mail, send your message to
the publisher at aphabooks@aphanet.org

Library of Congress Cataloging-in-Publication Data

Generali, Joyce A.
   The pharmacy technician's pocket drug reference / Joyce A. Generali.-2nd ed.
   p. cm.
   Includes index.
   ISBN 1-58212-048-X
   1. Pharmacy technicians—Handbooks, manuals, etc. 2. Drugs—
Handbooks, manuals, etc. I. Title: Pocket drug reference. II. American
Pharmaceutical Association. III. Title. [DNLM: 1 Pharmaceutical Preparations--
administration & dosage--Handbooks. 2. Pharmacists' Aides--Handbooks. QV
735 G326p 2002]

   RS122.95 .G464 2002
   615'.1—dc21

                                                           2002034301

HOW TO ORDER THIS BOOK
   Online: www.pharmacist.com
   By phone: 800-878-0729 (802-862-0095 from out-
   side the United States).
   VISA®, MasterCard®, and American Express® cards
   accepted

CONTENTS

Because the Food and Drug Administration (FDA) approves approximately 20 to 30 new chemical entities annually, keeping current with new drug products is a continuing concern for pharmacy technicians as well as pharmacists. *The Pharmacy Technician's Pocket Drug Reference* is the first drug information reference designed especially for pharmacy technicians to quickly identify drug products, their uses, and their dosage forms. The drugs included are categorized by generic names, trade names, therapeutic drug classes, general FDA approved therapeutic uses, and commercially available dosage forms.

Kept concise to foster quick and easy access, the book can be used at work or during study for examination. When more in-depth drug information is required, referral to other drug information resources and consultation with the supervising pharmacist are always recommended.

Although several brand names are listed for most generic drugs, please note that this is for identification purposes only and does not infer or imply therapeutic or generic equivalency. In addition, all dosage forms provided may not be available for every trade name listed.

Special care has been taken to include the top 200 most commonly prescribed drugs. In addition, most drugs marketed since 1997 have been included in an attempt to create a resource that would be useful in the practice setting.

Note that the information on most parenteral formulations is presented in final dose amounts of the container (e.g., syringe, vial, ampule) and not as the concentration of the drug. Amounts provided for parenteral formulations are not to be construed as appropriate doses. Some amounts are larger than typical doses because the container may be a multidose vial. This resource is not intended as a dosing guide and an appropriate resource should be consulted prior to patient care decisions.

I hope this is a useful addition to your library and optimizes the efficient and safe practice of pharmacy.

Joyce A. Generali, MS, RPh, FASHP
July 2002

ABBREVIATIONS

The following abbreviations are used in this book:

BPH—benign prostatic hyperplasia
CHF—congestive heart failure
CNS—central nervous system
GERD—gastroesophageal reflux disease
HCL—hydrochloride
HCTZ—hydrochlorothiazide
HIV—human immunodeficiency virus
IU—international units
LH—lutenizing hormone
LMWH—low molecular weight heparin
MI—myocardial infarction
MU—million units
NSAID—nonsteroidal anti-inflammatory drug
OTC—over-the-counter drug
PTCA—percutaneous transluminal coronary angioplasty

ABACAVIR

a BAK a veer

TRADE NAME(S):
Ziagen

THERAPEUTIC CLASS:
Antiviral

GENERAL USES:
HIV infection

DOSAGE FORMS:
Tablets: 300 mg;
Solution: 20 mg/mL

ABACAVIR/ LAMIVUDINE/ ZIDOVUDINE

a BAK a veer/ la MI vyoo deen/zye DOE vyoo deen

TRADE NAME(S):
Trizivir

THERAPEUTIC CLASS:
Antiviral

GENERAL USES:
HIV infection

DOSAGE FORMS:
Tablets: 300 mg/
150 mg/300 mg

ACARBOSE

AY car bose

TRADE NAME(S):
Precose

THERAPEUTIC CLASS:
Antidiabetic

GENERAL USES:
Diabetes (type 2)

DOSAGE FORMS:
Tablets: 25 mg, 50 mg,
100 mg

ACEBUTOLOL

a se BYOO toe lole

TRADE NAME(S):
Sectral

THERAPEUTIC CLASS:
Antihypertensive,
antiarrhythmic

GENERAL USES:
Hypertension, arrhyth-
mias

DOSAGE FORMS:
Capsules: 200 mg,
400 mg

ACETAMINOPHEN

a seet a MIN oh fen

TRADE NAME(S):
Tylenol, Tempra,
Aceta, many others

THERAPEUTIC CLASS:
Analgesic, antipyretic

GENERAL USES:
Pain, fever

DOSAGE FORMS:
Tablets: 160 mg, 325
mg, 500 mg, 650 mg;
Chewable tablets: 80
mg; Caplets: 160 mg,
500 mg, 650 mg;
Capsules: 325 mg,

500 mg; Drops: 80 mg/0.8 mL; Also Elixir, Liquid and Solution

ACETOHEXAMIDE
a set oh HEKS a mide
TRADE NAME(S):
Dymelor
THERAPEUTIC CLASS:
Antidiabetic
GENERAL USES:
Diabetes (type 2)
DOSAGE FORMS:
Tablets: 250 mg, 500 mg

ACITRETIN
ass ih TREH tin
TRADE NAME(S):
Soriatane
THERAPEUTIC CLASS:
Retinoid
GENERAL USES:
Psoriasis
DOSAGE FORMS:
Capsules: 10 mg, 25 mg

ACYCLOVIR
ay SYE kloe veer
TRADE NAME(S):
Zovirax
THERAPEUTIC CLASS:
Antiviral

GENERAL USES:
Herpes, shingles, chickenpox
DOSAGE FORMS:
Tablets: 400 mg, 800 mg; Capsules: 200 mg; Suspension: 200 mg/5 mL; Ointment: 5%; Injection: 500 mg, 1 g

ADAPALENE
a DAP a leen
TRADE NAME(S):
Differin
THERAPEUTIC CLASS:
Retinoid (topical)
GENERAL USES:
Acne vulgaris
DOSAGE FORMS:
Topical gel: 0.1%

ADEFOVIR DIPIVOXIL
a DEF o veer dye pi VOKS il
TRADE NAME(S):
Hepsera
THERAPEUTIC CLASS:
Antiviral
GENERAL USES:
Chronic hepatitis B
DOSAGE FORMS:
Tablets: 10 mg

ALBUTEROL
al BYOO ter ole
TRADE NAME(S):
Proventil, Ventolin,
Ventolin-HFA
THERAPEUTIC CLASS:
Bronchodilator
GENERAL USES:
Bronchospasm
DOSAGE FORMS:
Tablets: 2 mg, 4 mg;
Extended release
tablets: 4 mg, 8 mg;
Syrup: 2 mg/5 mL;
Aerosol: 90 mcg/
inhalation; Inhalation
solution: 0.083%,
0.5%; Inhalation cap-
sules: 200 mcg

ALCLOMETASONE
al kloe MET a sone
TRADE NAME(S):
Aclovate
THERAPEUTIC CLASS:
Corticosteroid
GENERAL USES:
Various skin conditions
DOSAGE FORMS:
Ointment & Cream:
0.05%

ALEMTUZUMAB
ay lem TU zoo mab

TRADE NAME(S):
Campath
THERAPEUTIC CLASS:
Monoclonal antibody
GENERAL USES:
Refractory leukemia
DOSAGE FORMS:
Injection: 30 mg

ALENDRONATE
a LEN droe nate
TRADE NAME(S):
Fosamax
THERAPEUTIC CLASS:
Bisphosphonate
GENERAL USES:
Osteoporosis, Paget's
disease
DOSAGE FORMS:
Tablets: 5 mg, 10 mg,
35 mg, 40 mg, 70 mg

ALITRETINOIN
a li TRET i noyn
TRADE NAME(S):
Panretin
THERAPEUTIC CLASS:
Retinoid (topical)
GENERAL USES:
Kaposi's sarcoma
cutaneous lesions
DOSAGE FORMS:
Topical gel: 0.1%

ALLOPURINOL
al oh PURE i nole
TRADE NAME(S):
Zyloprim
THERAPEUTIC CLASS:
Gout agent
GENERAL USES:
Gout, increased uric acid conditions, calcium stones
DOSAGE FORMS:
Tablets: 100 mg, 300 mg

ALMOTRIPTAN
al moh TRIP tan
TRADE NAME(S):
Axert
THERAPEUTIC CLASS:
Antimigraine agent
GENERAL USES:
Migraine treatment
DOSAGE FORMS:
Tablets: 6.25 mg, 12.5 mg

ALOSETRON
al OH seh trahn
TRADE NAME(S):
Lotronex
THERAPEUTIC CLASS:
Gastrointestinal agent
GENERAL USES:
Irritable bowel syndrome (women)

DOSAGE FORMS:
Tablets: 1 mg

ALPRAZOLAM
al PRAY zoe lam
TRADE NAME(S):
Xanax
THERAPEUTIC CLASS:
Antianxiety agent
GENERAL USES:
Anxiety, panic disorder
DOSAGE FORMS:
Tablets: 0.25 mg, 0.5 mg, 1 mg, 2 mg; Solution: 0.5 mg/5 mL, 1 mg/mL

ALTEPLASE
AL te plase
TRADE NAME(S):
Activase
THERAPEUTIC CLASS:
Thrombolytic agent
GENERAL USES:
Dissolves blood clots in MI, stroke, pulmonary embolism
DOSAGE FORMS:
Injection: 50 mg, 100 mg

AMANTADINE
a MAN ta deen
TRADE NAME(S):
Symmetrel
THERAPEUTIC CLASS:
Antiparkinson agent
GENERAL USES:
Parkinson's disease, drug induced extrapyramidal disorders
DOSAGE FORMS:
Tablets & Capsules: 100 mg; Syrup: 50 mg/5 mL

AMCINONIDE
am SIN oh nide
TRADE NAME(S):
Cyclocort
THERAPEUTIC CLASS:
Corticosteroid (topical)
GENERAL USES:
Various skin conditions
DOSAGE FORMS:
Ointment, Cream & Lotion: 0.1%

AMIKACIN
am i KAY sin
TRADE NAME(S):
Amikin
THERAPEUTIC CLASS:
Anti-infective
GENERAL USES:
Bacterial infections
DOSAGE FORMS:
Injection: 100 mg, 200 mg, 500 mg, 1 g

AMILORIDE
a MIL oh ride
TRADE NAME(S):
Midamor
THERAPEUTIC CLASS:
Diuretic
GENERAL USES:
CHF related edema, hypertension
DOSAGE FORMS:
Tablets: 5 mg

AMINOCAPROIC ACID
a mee noe ka PROE ik
TRADE NAME(S):
Amicar
THERAPEUTIC CLASS:
Hemostatic
GENERAL USES:
Excessive bleeding
DOSAGE FORMS:
Tablets: 500 mg; Syrup: 250 mg/mL

AMINOLEVULINIC ACID
a MEE noh lev yoo lin ik
TRADE NAME(S):
Levulan Kerastick

THERAPEUTIC CLASS:
Skin agent (topical)
GENERAL USES:
Precancerous skin
lesions on face or
scalp
DOSAGE FORMS:
Topical solution: 20%

AMINOPHYLLINE
am in AHF ih lin
TRADE NAME(S):
Phyllocontin
THERAPEUTIC CLASS:
Bronchodilator
GENERAL USES:
Asthma
DOSAGE FORMS: (equiva-
lent amount of theo-
phylline): Tablets: 100
mg (79 mg), 200 mg
(158 mg); Controlled
release tablets: 225
mg (178 mg); Oral liq-
uid: 105 mg/5 mL (90
mg/5 mL); Injection:
250 mg (197 mg), 500
mg (394 mg)

AMIODARONE
a MEE oh da rone
TRADE NAME(S):
Cordarone, Cordarone
IV, Pacerone
THERAPEUTIC CLASS:
Antiarrhythmic
GENERAL USES:
Ventricular arrhythmias
& fibrillation
DOSAGE FORMS:
Tablets: 200 mg;
Injection: 150 mg

AMITRIPTYLINE
a mee TRIP ti leen
TRADE NAME(S):
Elavil
THERAPEUTIC CLASS:
Antidepressant
GENERAL USES:
Depression
DOSAGE FORMS:
Tablets: 10 mg, 25
mg, 50 mg, 75 mg,
100 mg, 150 mg;
Injection: 100 mg

AMLODIPINE
am LOE di peen
TRADE NAME(S):
Norvasc
THERAPEUTIC CLASS:
Antihypertensive,
antianginal
GENERAL USES:
Hypertension, angina
DOSAGE FORMS:
Tablets: 2.5 mg, 5 mg,
10 mg

AMLODIPINE/ BENAZEPRIL

am LOE di peen/ben AY ze pril

TRADE NAME(S):
Lotrel

THERAPEUTIC CLASS:
Antihypertensive/ diuretic

GENERAL USES:
CHF, hypertension

DOSAGE FORMS:
Tablets: 2.5 mg/10 mg, 5 mg/10 mg, 5 mg/20 mg

AMOXAPINE

a MOKS a peen

TRADE NAME(S):
Asendin

THERAPEUTIC CLASS:
Antidepressant

GENERAL USES:
Depression

DOSAGE FORMS:
Tablets: 25 mg, 50 mg, 100 mg, 150 mg

AMOXICILLIN

a moks i SIL in

TRADE NAME(S):
Amoxil, Trimox, Wymox

THERAPEUTIC CLASS:
Anti-infective

GENERAL USES:
Bacterial infections

DOSAGE FORMS:
Chewable tablets: 125 mg, 200 mg, 250 mg, 400 mg; Tablets: 500 mg, 875 mg; Capsules: 250 mg, 500 mg; Suspension: 50 mg/mL, 125 mg/5 mL, 200 mg/5 mL, 250 mg/5 mL, 400 mg/5 mL

AMOXICILLIN/ CLAVULANATE

a moks i SIL in/klav yoo LAN ate

TRADE NAME(S):
Augmentin, Augmentin ES

THERAPEUTIC CLASS:
Anti-infective

GENERAL USES:
Bacterial infections

DOSAGE FORMS:
Tablets: 250 mg/125 mg, 500 mg/125 mg, 875 mg/125 mg; Chewable tablets & suspension (per 5 mL): 125 mg/31.25 mg, 200 mg/28.5 mg, 250 mg/62.5 mg, 400 mg/57 mg; High dose suspension:

600 mg/42.9 mg (per 5 mL)

AMPHOTERICIN B (ORAL)

am foe TER i sin bee

TRADE NAME(S):
Fungizone

THERAPEUTIC CLASS:
Antifungal

GENERAL USES:
Oral fungal infection (candidiasis)

DOSAGE FORMS:
Suspension: 100 mg/mL; Cream, Lotion & Ointment: 3%

AMPHOTERICIN B DESOXYCHOLATE (NONLIPID BASED)

am foe TER i sin bee des oks ee KOE late

TRADE NAME(S):
Fungizone, Amphocin

THERAPEUTIC CLASS:
Antifungal

GENERAL USES:
Systemic fungal infections

DOSAGE FORMS:
Injection: 50 mg

AMPHOTERICIN B, LIPID BASED

am foe TER i sin bee

TRADE NAME(S):
Abelcet, Amphotec, AmBisome

THERAPEUTIC CLASS:
Antifungal

GENERAL USES:
Systemic fungal infections

DOSAGE FORMS:
Injection: 50 mg, 100 mg

AMPICILLIN

am pi SIL in

TRADE NAME(S):
Principen, Omnipen, Totacillin

THERAPEUTIC CLASS:
Anti-infective

GENERAL USES:
Bacterial infections

DOSAGE FORMS:
Capsules: 250 mg, 500 mg; Suspension: 125 mg/5 mL, 250 mg/5 mL; Injection: 125 mg, 250 mg, 500 mg, 1 g, 2 g, 10 g

AMPICILLIN SODIUM/ SULBACTAM SODIUM

am pi SIL in/SUL bak tam

TRADE NAME(S):
Unasyn

THERAPEUTIC CLASS:
Anti-infective

GENERAL USES:
Bacterial infections

DOSAGE FORMS:
Injection: 1 g/0.5 g, 2 g/1 g, 10 g/5 g

AMPRENAVIR

am PREN a veer

TRADE NAME(S):
Agenerase

THERAPEUTIC CLASS:
Antiviral

GENERAL USES:
HIV infection

DOSAGE FORMS:
Capsules: 50 mg, 150 mg; Solution: 15 mg/mL

ANAGRELIDE

an AG gre lide

TRADE NAME(S):
Agrylin

THERAPEUTIC CLASS:
Antiplatelet agent

GENERAL USES:
Essential thrombocy-topenia

DOSAGE FORMS:
Capsules: 0.5 mg, 1 mg

ANAKINRA

an a KIN ra

TRADE NAME(S):
Kineret

THERAPEUTIC CLASS:
Biological

GENERAL USES:
Rheumatoid arthritis

DOSAGE FORMS:
Injection: 100 mg

ANASTROZOLE

an AS troe zole

TRADE NAME(S):
Arimidex

THERAPEUTIC CLASS:
Antineoplastic

GENERAL USES:
Breast cancer

DOSAGE FORMS:
Tablets: 1 mg

ANTHRALIN

AN thra lin

TRADE NAME(S):
Anthra-Derm, Drithocreme

THERAPEUTIC CLASS:
Antipsoriatic (topical)

GENERAL USES:
Psoriasis
DOSAGE FORMS:
Ointment & Cream:
0.1%, 0.25%, 0.4%,
0.5%, 1%; Cream: 0.2%

APRACLONIDINE
a pra KLOE ni deen
TRADE NAME(S):
Iopidine
THERAPEUTIC CLASS:
Ocular agent
GENERAL USES:
Decrease intraocular
pressure
DOSAGE FORMS:
Ophthalmic solution:
0.5%, 1%

ARGATROBAN
ar GA troh ban
TRADE NAME(S):
Acova
THERAPEUTIC CLASS:
Anticoagulant
GENERAL USES:
Anticoagulation in
hemodialysis
DOSAGE FORMS:
Injection: 250 mg

ARSENIC TRIOXIDE
AR se nik tri OKS id

TRADE NAME(S):
Trisenox
THERAPEUTIC CLASS:
Antineoplastic
GENERAL USES:
Acute promyelocytic
leukemia
DOSAGE FORMS:
Injection: 10 mg

ASPIRIN
AS pir in
TRADE NAME(S):
Empirin, ZORprin,
many others
THERAPEUTIC CLASS:
Analgesic, antipyretic,
anti-inflammatory
GENERAL USES:
Pain, fever (adults),
arthritis
DOSAGE FORMS:
Tablets: 81 mg, 165 mg,
325 mg, 500 mg, 650
mg, 975 mg; Extended
release tablets: 650 mg,
800 mg

ASPIRIN/
DIPYRIDAMOLE
AS pir in/dye peer ID a
mole
TRADE NAME(S):
Aggrenox
THERAPEUTIC CLASS:

Antithrombotic
GENERAL USES:
Reduce stroke risk
DOSAGE FORMS:
Capsules: 25 mg/200 mg

ATENOLOL
a TEN oh lole
TRADE NAME(S):
Tenormin
THERAPEUTIC CLASS:
Cardiac agent
GENERAL USES:
Hypertension
DOSAGE FORMS:
Tablets: 25 mg, 50 mg, 100 mg; Injection: 5 mg

ATENOLOL/ CHLORTHALIDONE
a TEN oh lole/klor THAL i done
TRADE NAME(S):
Tenoretic
THERAPEUTIC CLASS:
Antihypertensive/ diuretic
GENERAL USES:
Hypertension
DOSAGE FORMS:
Tablets: 100 mg/25 mg, 50 mg/25 mg

ATORVASTATIN
a TORE va sta tin
TRADE NAME(S):
Lipitor
THERAPEUTIC CLASS:
Antilipemic
GENERAL USES:
Hyperlipidemia, hyper-triglyceridemia
DOSAGE FORMS:
Tablets: 10 mg, 20 mg, 40 mg, 80 mg

ATOVAQUONE/ PROGUANIL
a TOE va kwone/pro GWA nil
TRADE NAME(S):
Malarone, Malarone-Pediatric
THERAPEUTIC CLASS:
Antimalarial
GENERAL USES:
Malaria treatment and prevention
DOSAGE FORMS:
Tablets: 250 mg/100 mg, 62.5 mg/25 mg

ATROPINE
A troe peen
TRADE NAME(S):
Isopto Atropine
THERAPEUTIC CLASS:
Ocular agent

GENERAL USES:
Pupil dilation
DOSAGE FORMS:
Ophthalmic solution:
0.5%, 1%, 2%;
Ophthalmic ointment: 1%

AURANOFIN
au RANE oh fin
TRADE NAME(S):
Ridaura
THERAPEUTIC CLASS:
Antirheumatic agent
GENERAL USES:
Rheumatoid arthritis
DOSAGE FORMS:
Capsules: 3 mg

AZATADINE
a ZA ta deen
TRADE NAME(S):
Optimine
THERAPEUTIC CLASS:
Antihistamine
GENERAL USES:
Allergic rhinitis/hives
DOSAGE FORMS:
Tablets: 1 mg

AZITHROMYCIN
az ith roe MYE sin
TRADE NAME(S):
Zithromax

THERAPEUTIC CLASS:
Anti-infective
GENERAL USES:
Bacterial infections
DOSAGE FORMS:
Tablets: 250 mg, 600
mg; Suspension: 100
mg/5 mL, 200 mg/5
mL; Injection: 500 mg

AZTREONAM
AZ tree oh nam
TRADE NAME(S):
Azactam
THERAPEUTIC CLASS:
Anti-infective
GENERAL USES:
Bacterial infections
DOSAGE FORMS:
Injection: 500 mg, 1 g,
2 g

BACAMPICILLIN
ba cam pih SILL in
TRADE NAME(S):
Spectrobid
THERAPEUTIC CLASS:
Anti-infective
GENERAL USES:
Bacterial infections
DOSAGE FORMS:
Tablets: 400 mg

BACITRACIN
bas i TRAY sin
TRADE NAME(S):
  AK-Tracin
THERAPEUTIC CLASS:
  Ocular agent (anti-infective)
GENERAL USES:
  Ocular infections
DOSAGE FORMS:
  Ophthalmic ointment: 500 u/g

BACLOFEN
BAK loe fen
TRADE NAME(S):
  Lioresal, Lioresal Intrathecal
THERAPEUTIC CLASS:
  Skeletal muscle relaxant
GENERAL USES:
  Spasticity
DOSAGE FORMS:
  Tablets: 10 mg, 20 mg; Injection: 0.05 mg, 0.5 mg, 2 mg

BALSALAZIDE
bal SAL a zide
TRADE NAME(S):
  Colazal
THERAPEUTIC CLASS:
  Gastrointestinal agent

GENERAL USES:
  Ulcerative colitis
DOSAGE FORMS:
  Capsules: 750 mg

BECAPLERMIN
be KAP ler min
TRADE NAME(S):
  Regranex
THERAPEUTIC CLASS:
  Wound healer (topical)
GENERAL USES:
  Diabetic neuropathic ulcers
DOSAGE FORMS:
  Topical gel: 0.01%

BECLOMETHASONE (INHALED)
be kloe METH a sone
TRADE NAME(S):
  Vanceril, Beclovent, Qvar
THERAPEUTIC CLASS:
  Corticosteroid (inhaler)
GENERAL USES:
  Asthma (chronic)
DOSAGE FORMS:
  Inhaler: 40 mcg/inhalation, 42 mcg/inhalation, 80 mcg/inhalation, 84 mcg/inhalation

BECLOMETHASONE (NASAL)

be kloe METH a sone

TRADE NAME(S):
Beconase, Vancenase, Beconase AQ, Vancenase AQ

THERAPEUTIC CLASS:
Corticosteroid (nasal)

GENERAL USES:
Allergies

DOSAGE FORMS:
Nasal spray: 0.042%, 0.084%

BENAZEPRIL

ben AY ze pril

TRADE NAME(S):
Lotensin

THERAPEUTIC CLASS:
Antihypertensive

GENERAL USES:
Hypertension

DOSAGE FORMS:
Tablets: 5 mg, 10 mg, 20 mg, 40 mg

BENAZEPRIL/HCTZ

ben AY ze pril/hye droe klor oh THYE a zide

TRADE NAME(S):
Lotensin HCT

THERAPEUTIC CLASS:
Antihypertensive/diuretic

GENERAL USES:
Hypertension

DOSAGE FORMS:
Tablets: 5 mg/6.25 mg, 10 mg/12.5 mg, 20 mg/12.5 mg, 20 mg/25 mg

BENZONATATE

ben ZOE na tate

TRADE NAME(S):
Tessalon Perles

THERAPEUTIC CLASS:
Nonnarcotic cough suppressant

GENERAL USES:
Relief of cough

DOSAGE FORMS:
Capsules: 100 mg

BENZOYL PEROXIDE

BEN zoe il peer OKS ide

TRADE NAME(S):
Benzac, Peroxin, Persa-Gel, many others

THERAPEUTIC CLASS:
Anti-infective (topical)

GENERAL USES:
Acne

DOSAGE FORMS:
Liquid, Lotion, Cream, Gel: 2.5%, 5%, 10%

BENZTROPINE

BENZ troe peen

TRADE NAME(S):
Cogentin

THERAPEUTIC CLASS:
Antiparkinson agent

GENERAL USES:
Parkinson's disease, drug induced extrapyramidal disorders

DOSAGE FORMS:
Tablets: 0.5 mg, 1 mg, 2 mg

BEPRIDIL

BE pri dil

TRADE NAME(S):
Vascor

THERAPEUTIC CLASS:
Antianginal

GENERAL USES:
Angina

DOSAGE FORMS:
Tablets: 200 mg, 300 mg, 400 mg

BETAMETHASONE DIPROPRIONATE

bay ta METH a sone

TRADE NAME(S):
Diprosone, Alphatrex, Maxivate

THERAPEUTIC CLASS:
Corticosteroid (topical)

GENERAL USES:
Various skin conditions

DOSAGE FORMS:
Ointment, Cream & Lotion: 0.05%; Aerosol: 0.1%

BETAMETHASONE VALERATE

bay ta METH a sone

TRADE NAME(S):
Betatrex, Valisone

THERAPEUTIC CLASS:
Corticosteroid (topical)

GENERAL USES:
Various skin conditions

DOSAGE FORMS:
Ointment, Cream & Lotion: 0.1%; Cream: 0.01%, 0.05%

BETAXOLOL (OCULAR)

be TAKS oh lol

TRADE NAME(S):
Betoptic, Betoptic S

THERAPEUTIC CLASS:
Ocular agent

GENERAL USES:
Glaucoma/ocular hypertension

DOSAGE FORMS:
Ophthalmic solution: 0.5%; Ophthalmic suspension: 0.25%

BETAXOLOL (ORAL)
be TAKS oh lol
TRADE NAME(S):
Kerlone
THERAPEUTIC CLASS:
Antihypertensive
GENERAL USES:
Hypertension
DOSAGE FORMS:
Tablets: 10 mg, 20 mg

BEXAROTENE
beks AIR oh teen
TRADE NAME(S):
Targretin
THERAPEUTIC CLASS:
Antineoplastic
GENERAL USES:
T-cell lymphoma
DOSAGE FORMS:
Capsules: 75 mg

BICALUTAMIDE
bye ka LOO ta mide
TRADE NAME(S):
Casodex
THERAPEUTIC CLASS:
Antiandrogen antineo-
plastic
GENERAL USES:
Prostate cancer
DOSAGE FORMS:
Tablets: 50 mg

BIMATOPROST
bi MAT oh prost
TRADE NAME(S):
Lumigan
THERAPEUTIC CLASS:
Ocular agent
GENERAL USES:
Ocular hypertension
DOSAGE FORMS:
Ophthalmic solution:
0.03%

BIPERIDEN
by PURR ih den
TRADE NAME(S):
Akineton
THERAPEUTIC CLASS:
Antiparkinson agent
GENERAL USES:
Parkinson's disease,
drug induced
extrapyramidal disor-
ders
DOSAGE FORMS:
Tablets: 2 mg

BISOPROLOL
bis OH proe lol
TRADE NAME(S):
Zebeta
THERAPEUTIC CLASS:
Antihypertensive
GENERAL USES:
Hypertension

DOSAGE FORMS:
  Tablets: 5 mg, 10 mg

BISOPROLOL/HCTZ
bis OH proe lol/hye droe
klor oh THYE a zide
TRADE NAME(S):
  Ziac
THERAPEUTIC CLASS:
  Antihypertensive/diur-
  etic
GENERAL USES:
  Hypertension
DOSAGE FORMS:
  Tablets: 2.5 mg/6.25
  mg, 5 mg/6.25 mg, 10
  mg/6.25 mg

BITOLTEROL
bye TOLE ter ole
TRADE NAME(S):
  Tornalate
THERAPEUTIC CLASS:
  Bronchodilator
GENERAL USES:
  Bronchospasm/asth-
  ma
DOSAGE FORMS:
  Inhalation solution:
  0.2%; Aerosol: 0.8%

BIVALIRUDIN
bye VAL i roo din
TRADE NAME(S):
  Angiomax
THERAPEUTIC CLASS:
  Anticoagulant
GENERAL USES:
  Prevention of clotting
  in angina/PTCA
DOSAGE FORMS:
  Injection: 250 mg

BOSENTAN
boe SEN tan
TRADE NAME(S):
  Tracleer
THERAPEUTIC CLASS:
  Cardiac agent
GENERAL USES:
  Pulmonary hyperten-
  sion
DOSAGE FORMS:
  Tablets: 62.5 mg,
  125 mg

BOTULINUM TOXIN TYPE A
BOT yoo lin num TOKS in
TRADE NAME(S):
  Botox
THERAPEUTIC CLASS:
  Toxoid
GENERAL USES:
  Cervical dystonia,
  facial wrinkles
DOSAGE FORMS:
  Injection: 100 units

BOTULINUM TOXIN TYPE B

BOT yoo lin num TOKS in

TRADE NAME(S):
Myobloc

THERAPEUTIC CLASS:
Toxoid

GENERAL USES:
Cervical dystonia

DOSAGE FORMS:
Injection: 2500 units, 5000 units, 10,000 units

BRIMONIDINE

bri MOE ni deen

TRADE NAME(S):
Alphagan, Alphagan-P

THERAPEUTIC CLASS:
Ocular agent

GENERAL USES:
Glaucoma/ocular hypertension

DOSAGE FORMS:
Ophthalmic solution: 0.15%, 0.2%

BRINZOLAMIDE

brin ZOH la mide

TRADE NAME(S):
Azopt

THERAPEUTIC CLASS:
Ocular agent

GENERAL USES:
Glaucoma/ocular hypertension

DOSAGE FORMS:
Ophthalmic solution: 1%

BROMOCRIPTINE

broe moe KRIP teen

TRADE NAME(S):
Parlodel

THERAPEUTIC CLASS:
Antiparkinson agent

GENERAL USES:
Parkinson's disease

DOSAGE FORMS:
Tablets: 2.5 mg; Capsules: 5 mg

BUDESONIDE

byoo DES oh nide

TRADE NAME(S):
Entocort EC

THERAPEUTIC CLASS:
Corticosteroid

GENERAL USES:
Crohn's disease

DOSAGE FORMS:
Capsules: 3 mg

BUDESONIDE (INHALED)

byoo DES oh nide

TRADE NAME(S):
Pulmicort
THERAPEUTIC CLASS:
Corticosteroid (inhaler)
GENERAL USES:
Asthma (chronic)
DOSAGE FORMS:
Inhaler: 200
mcg/inhalation;
Inhalation suspension:
0.25 mg/2 mL, 0.5
mg/2 mL

BUDESONIDE
(NASAL)
byoo DES oh nide
TRADE NAME(S):
Rhinocort, Rhinocort
Aqua
THERAPEUTIC CLASS:
Corticosteroid (nasal)
GENERAL USES:
Allergies
DOSAGE FORMS:
Nasal aerosol: 32
mcg/spray

BUMETANIDE
byoo MET a nide
TRADE NAME(S):
Bumex
THERAPEUTIC CLASS:
Diuretic
GENERAL USES:
CHF related edema,

hypertension
DOSAGE FORMS:
Tablets: 0.5 mg,
1 mg, 2 mg; Injection:
0.5 mg, 1 mg, 2.5 mg

BUPROPION
byoo PROE pee on
TRADE NAME(S):
Wellbutrin, Wellbutrin
SR
THERAPEUTIC CLASS:
Antidepressant
GENERAL USES:
Depression
DOSAGE FORMS:
Tablets: 75 mg,
100 mg; Sustained
release tablets: 100
mg, 150 mg

BUPROPION
byoo PROE pee on
TRADE NAME(S):
Zyban
THERAPEUTIC CLASS:
Smoking deterrent
GENERAL USES:
Smoking cessation
DOSAGE FORMS:
Sustained release
tablets: 150 mg

BUSPIRONE
byoo SPYE rone
Trade name(s):
BuSpar
Therapeutic Class:
Antidepressant
General Uses:
Depression
Dosage Forms:
Tablets: 5 mg, 10 mg,
15 mg, 30 mg

BUTABARBITAL
byoo ta BAR bi tal
Trade name(s):
Butisol
Therapeutic Class:
Sedative/hypnotic
General Uses:
Insomnia (short term
therapy)
Dosage Forms:
Tablets: 15 mg,
30 mg, 50 mg, 100
mg; Elixir: 30 mg/5 mL

BUTENAFINE
byoo TEN a feen
Trade name(s):
Mentax
Therapeutic Class:
Antifungal (topical)
General Uses:
Athlete's foot

Dosage Forms:
Cream: 1%

CABERGOLINE
ca BER goe leen
Trade name(s):
Dostinex
Therapeutic Class:
Dopamine receptor
agonist
General Uses:
Hyperprolactinemia
Dosage Forms:
Tablets: 0.5 mg

CALCIPOTRIENE
kal si POE try een
Trade name(s):
Dovonex
Therapeutic Class:
Antipsoriatic (topical)
General Uses:
Psoriasis
Dosage Forms:
Ointment, Solution &
Cream: 0.005%

CALCIUM CHLORIDE
KAL see um KLOR ide
Trade name(s):
Calcium Chloride
Therapeutic Class:
Electrolyte

GENERAL USES:
  Replacement
DOSAGE FORMS:
  Injection: 10%

CALCIUM GLUCONATE
KAL see um GLOO koe
nate
TRADE NAME(S):
  Calcium Gluconate
THERAPEUTIC CLASS:
  Electrolyte
GENERAL USES:
  Replacement
DOSAGE FORMS:
  Injection: 10%

CANDESARTAN
kan de SAR tan
TRADE NAME(S):
  Atacand
THERAPEUTIC CLASS:
  Antihypertensive
GENERAL USES:
  Hypertension
DOSAGE FORMS:
  Tablets: 4 mg, 8 mg,
  16 mg, 32 mg

CAPECITABINE
ka pe SITE a been
TRADE NAME(S):
  Xeloda

THERAPEUTIC CLASS:
  Antineoplastic
GENERAL USES:
  Metastatic breast cancer
DOSAGE FORMS:
  Tablets: 150 mg,
  500 mg

CAPTOPRIL
KAP toe pril
TRADE NAME(S):
  Capoten
THERAPEUTIC CLASS:
  Antihypertensive,
  cardiac agent
GENERAL USES:
  Hypertension, heart
  failure, left ventricular
  dysfunction, diabetic
  renal dysfunction
DOSAGE FORMS:
  Tablets: 12.5 mg,
  25 mg, 50 mg, 100
  mg

CAPTOPRIL/HCTZ
KAP toe pril/hye droe
klor oh THYE a zide
TRADE NAME(S):
  Capozide
THERAPEUTIC CLASS:
  Antihypertensive/diuretic
GENERAL USES:
  Hypertension

DOSAGE FORMS:
Tablets: 25 mg/15 mg,
50 mg/15 mg,
25 mg/25 mg,
50 mg/25 mg

CARBAMAZEPINE
kar ba MAZ e peen
TRADE NAME(S):
Tegretol, Epitol
THERAPEUTIC CLASS:
Anticonvulsant
GENERAL USES:
Seizures, trigeminal
neuralgia
DOSAGE FORMS:
Chewable tablets: 100
mg; Tablets: 200 mg;
Extended release
tablets: 100 mg, 200
mg, 400 mg;
Extended release cap-
sules: 200 mg, 300
mg; Suspension: 100
mg/5 mL

CARBENICILLIN
kar ben i SIL in
TRADE NAME(S):
Geocillin
THERAPEUTIC CLASS:
Anti-infective
GENERAL USES:
Bacterial infections

DOSAGE FORMS:
Tablets: 382 mg

CARISOPRODOL
kar eye soe PROE dole
TRADE NAME(S):
Soma
THERAPEUTIC CLASS:
Skeletal muscle relaxant
GENERAL USES:
Musculoskeletal condi-
tions
DOSAGE FORMS:
Tablets: 350 mg

CARTEOLOL (OCULAR)
KAR tee oh lole
TRADE NAME(S):
Ocupress
THERAPEUTIC CLASS:
Ocular agent
GENERAL USES:
Glaucoma/ocular
hypertension
DOSAGE FORMS:
Ophthalmic solution:
1%

CARTEOLOL (ORAL)
KAR tee oh lole
TRADE NAME(S):
Cartrol
THERAPEUTIC CLASS:
Antihypertensive

GENERAL USES:
Hypertension
DOSAGE FORMS:
Tablets: 2.5 mg, 5 mg

CARVEDILOL
KAR ve dil ole
TRADE NAME(S):
Coreg
THERAPEUTIC CLASS:
Antihypertensive,
cardiac agent
GENERAL USES:
Hypertension, congestive heart failure
DOSAGE FORMS:
Tablets: 3.125 mg, 6.25
mg, 12.5 mg, 25 mg

CASPOFUNGIN ACETATE
kas poe FUN jin
TRADE NAME(S):
Cancidas
THERAPEUTIC CLASS:
Antifungal
GENERAL USES:
Refractory aspergillosis
infection
DOSAGE FORMS:
Injection: 50 mg, 70 mg

CEFACLOR
SEF a klor
TRADE NAME(S):
Ceclor
THERAPEUTIC CLASS:
Anti-infective
GENERAL USES:
Bacterial infections
DOSAGE FORMS:
Capsules: 250 mg,
500 mg; Extended
release tablets:
375 mg, 500 mg;
Suspension: 125 mg/
5 mL, 187 mg/5 mL,
250 mg/5 mL,
375 mg/5 mL

CEFADROXIL
sef a DROKS il
TRADE NAME(S):
Duricef
THERAPEUTIC CLASS:
Anti-infective
GENERAL USES:
Bacterial infections
DOSAGE FORMS:
Capsules: 500 mg;
Tablets: 1 g;
Suspension: 125 mg/
5 mL, 250 mg/
5 mL, 500 mg/5 mL

CEFAMANDOLE
sef a MAN dole
TRADE NAME(S):
  Mandol
THERAPEUTIC CLASS:
  Anti-infective
GENERAL USES:
  Bacterial infections
DOSAGE FORMS:
  Injection: 1 g, 2 g

CEFAZOLIN
sef A zoe lin
TRADE NAME(S):
  Ancef, Kefzol
THERAPEUTIC CLASS:
  Anti-infective
GENERAL USES:
  Bacterial infections
DOSAGE FORMS:
  Injection: 250 mg, 500
  mg, 1 g, 5 g, 10 g, 20 g

CEFDINIR
SEF di ner
TRADE NAME(S):
  Omnicef
THERAPEUTIC CLASS:
  Anti-infective
GENERAL USES:
  Bacterial infections
DOSAGE FORMS:
  Capsules: 300 mg;
  Suspension: 125 mg/
  5 mL

CEFDITOREN PIVOXIL
sef da TOR en
pye VOKS il
TRADE NAME(S):
  Spectracef
THERAPEUTIC CLASS:
  Anti-infective
GENERAL USES:
  Bacterial infections
DOSAGE FORMS:
  Tablets: 200 mg

CEFEPIME
SEF e pim
TRADE NAME(S):
  Maxipime
THERAPEUTIC CLASS:
  Anti-infective
GENERAL USES:
  Bacterial infections
DOSAGE FORMS:
  Injection: 500 mg, 1 g,
  2 g

CEFIXIME
sef IKS eem
TRADE NAME(S):
  Suprax
THERAPEUTIC CLASS:
  Anti-infective
GENERAL USES:
  Bacterial infections

DOSAGE FORMS:
Tablets: 200 mg, 400 mg; Suspension: 100 mg/5 mL

CEFMETAZOLE
seff MET ah zole
TRADE NAME(S):
Zefazone
THERAPEUTIC CLASS:
Anti-infective
GENERAL USES:
Bacterial infections
DOSAGE FORMS:
Injection: 1 g, 2 g

CEFONICID
se FAHN ih sid
TRADE NAME(S):
Monocid
THERAPEUTIC CLASS:
Anti-infective
GENERAL USES:
Bacterial infections
DOSAGE FORMS:
Injection: 1 g, 10 g

CEFOPERAZONE
sef oh PER a zone
TRADE NAME(S):
Cefobid
THERAPEUTIC CLASS:
Anti-infective
GENERAL USES:

Bacterial infections
DOSAGE FORMS:
Injection: 1 g, 2 g, 10 g

CEFOTAXIME SODIUM
sef oh TAKS eem
TRADE NAME(S):
Claforan
THERAPEUTIC CLASS:
Anti-infective
GENERAL USES:
Bacterial infections
DOSAGE FORMS:
Injection: 500 mg, 1 g, 2 g, 10 g

CEFOTETAN DISODIUM
SEF oh tee tan
TRADE NAME(S):
Cefotan
THERAPEUTIC CLASS:
Anti-infective
GENERAL USES:
Bacterial infections
DOSAGE FORMS:
Injection: 1 g, 2 g, 10 g

CEFOXITIN SODIUM
se FOKS i tin
TRADE NAME(S):
Mefoxin
THERAPEUTIC CLASS:
Anti-infective
GENERAL USES:

Bacterial infections
DOSAGE FORMS:
Injection: 1 g, 2 g, 10 g

CEFPODOXIME
sef pode OKS eem
TRADE NAME(S):
Vantin
THERAPEUTIC CLASS:
Anti-infective
GENERAL USES:
Bacterial infections
DOSAGE FORMS:
Tablets: 100 mg,
200 mg; Suspension:
50 mg/5 mL,
100 mg/5 mL

CEFPROZIL
sef PROE zil
TRADE NAME(S):
Cefzil
THERAPEUTIC CLASS:
Anti-infective
GENERAL USES:
Bacterial infections
DOSAGE FORMS:
Capsules: 250 mg,
500 mg; Suspension:
125 mg/5 mL,
250 mg/5 mL

CEFTAZIDIME
SEF tay zi deem

TRADE NAME(S):
Fortaz, Ceptaz,
Tazidime
THERAPEUTIC CLASS:
Anti-infective
GENERAL USES:
Bacterial infections
DOSAGE FORMS:
Injection: 500 mg, 1 g,
2 g, 6 g, 10 g

CEFTIBUTEN
sef TYE byoo ten
TRADE NAME(S):
Cedax
THERAPEUTIC CLASS:
Anti-infective
GENERAL USES:
Bacterial infections
DOSAGE FORMS:
Capsules: 400 mg;
Suspension: 90 mg/5
mL, 180 mg/5 mL

CEFTIZOXIME SODIUM
sef ti ZOKS eem
TRADE NAME(S):
Cefizox
THERAPEUTIC CLASS:
Anti-infective
GENERAL USES:
Bacterial infections
DOSAGE FORMS:
Injection: 500 mg, 1 g,
2 g, 10 g

CEFTRIAXONE SODIUM

sef trye AKS one

TRADE NAME(S):
Rocephin

THERAPEUTIC CLASS:
Anti-infective

GENERAL USES:
Bacterial infections

DOSAGE FORMS:
Injection: 250 mg, 500 mg, 1 g, 2 g, 10 g

CEFUROXIME

se fyoor OKS eem

TRADE NAME(S):
Ceftin

THERAPEUTIC CLASS:
Anti-infective

GENERAL USES:
Bacterial infections

DOSAGE FORMS:
Tablets: 125 mg, 250 mg, 500 mg; Suspension: 125 mg/5 mL, 250 mg/5 mL; Injection: 750 mg, 1.5 g, 7.5 g

CELECOXIB

se le KOKS ib

TRADE NAME(S):
Celebrex

THERAPEUTIC CLASS:
Anti-inflammatory/ analgesic

GENERAL USES:
Osteoarthritis, rheumatoid arthritis

DOSAGE FORMS:
Capsules: 100 mg, 200 mg

CEPHALEXIN

sef a LEKS in

TRADE NAME(S):
Keflex, Biocef

THERAPEUTIC CLASS:
Anti-infective

GENERAL USES:
Bacterial infections

DOSAGE FORMS:
Capsules: 250 mg, 500 mg; Tablets: 250 mg, 500 mg; Suspension: 125 mg/5 mL, 250 mg/5 mL

CEPHALEXIN HYDROCHLORIDE

sef a LEKS in

TRADE NAME(S):
Keftab

THERAPEUTIC CLASS:
Anti-infective

GENERAL USES:
Bacterial infections

DOSAGE FORMS:
Tablets: 500 mg

CEPHRADINE
SEF ra deen
TRADE NAME(S):
Velosef
THERAPEUTIC CLASS:
Anti-infective
GENERAL USES:
Bacterial infections
DOSAGE FORMS:
Capsules: 250 mg,
500 mg; Suspension:
125 mg/5 mL, 250
mg/5 mL; Injection:
250 mg, 500 mg, 1 g,
2 g

CETIRIZINE
se TI ra zeen
TRADE NAME(S):
Zyrtec
THERAPEUTIC CLASS:
Antihistamine
GENERAL USES:
Allergic rhinitis/hives
DOSAGE FORMS:
Tablets: 5 mg, 10 mg;
Syrup: 5 mg/5 mL

CETRORELIX ACETATE
set roe REL iks
TRADE NAME(S):
Cetrotide
THERAPEUTIC CLASS:
Hormone antagonist
GENERAL USES:
Prevention of LH
surges
DOSAGE FORMS:
Injection: 0.25 mg, 3 mg

CEVIMELINE
se vi ME leen
TRADE NAME(S):
Evoxac
THERAPEUTIC CLASS:
Saliva stimulant
GENERAL USES:
Dry mouth in Sjögren's
syndrome
DOSAGE FORMS:
Capsules: 30 mg

CHLORAL HYDRATE
KLOR al HYE drate
TRADE NAME(S):
Aquachloral
Supprettes
THERAPEUTIC CLASS:
Sedative/hypnotic
GENERAL USES:
Pre-op sedation
DOSAGE FORMS:
Capsules: 500 mg;
Syrup: 250 mg/5 mL,
500 mg/5 mL

CHLORAMPHENICOL (OCULAR)

klor am FEN i kole

TRADE NAME(S):
AK-Chlor, Chloroptic, Ocuchlor

THERAPEUTIC CLASS:
Ocular agent (anti-infective)

GENERAL USES:
Ocular infections

DOSAGE FORMS:
Ophthalmic solution: 5 mg/mL; Ophthalmic ointment: 10 mg/g

CHLORAMPHENICOL (ORAL)

klor am FEN i kole

TRADE NAME(S):
Chloromycetin

THERAPEUTIC CLASS:
Anti-infective

GENERAL USES:
Bacterial infections

DOSAGE FORMS:
Capsules: 250 mg; Injection: 1 g

CHLORDIAZEPOXIDE

klor dye az e POKS ide

TRADE NAME(S):
Librium, Mitran, Libritabs

THERAPEUTIC CLASS:
Antianxiety agent, anti-convulsant

GENERAL USES:
Anxiety, alcohol withdrawal, seizures

DOSAGE FORMS:
Capsules: 5 mg, 10 mg, 25 mg; Tablets: 10 mg, 25 mg; Injection: 100 mg

CHLORDIAZEPOXIDE/ AMITRIPTYLINE

klor dye az e POKS ide/a mee TRIP ti leen

TRADE NAME(S):
Limbitrol DS

THERAPEUTIC CLASS:
Sedative/antidepressant

GENERAL USES:
Depression/anxiety

DOSAGE FORMS:
Tablets: 5 mg/12.5 mg, 10 mg/25 mg

CHLOROQUINE PHOSPHATE

KLOR oh kwin

TRADE NAME(S):
Aralen

THERAPEUTIC CLASS:
Antimalarial

GENERAL USES:
Malaria treatment and

prevention, intestinal
amebiasis
DOSAGE FORMS:
Tablets: 250 mg,
500 mg

mg, 75 mg, 150 mg,
200 mg, 300 mg;
Syrup: 10 mg/5 mL;
Concentrated solution:
30 mg/mL, 100
mg/mL; Injection:
25 mg, 50 mg

CHLOROTHIAZIDE
klor oh THYE a zide
TRADE NAME(S):
Diuril
THERAPEUTIC CLASS:
Diuretic
GENERAL USES:
CHF related edema,
hypertension
DOSAGE FORMS:
Tablets: 250 mg,
500 mg; Suspension:
250 mg/5 mL

CHLORPROPAMIDE
klor PROE pa mide
TRADE NAME(S):
Diabinese
THERAPEUTIC CLASS:
Antidiabetic
GENERAL USES:
Diabetes (type 2)
DOSAGE FORMS:
Tablets: 100 mg,
250 mg

CHLORPROMAZINE
klor PROE ma zeen
TRADE NAME(S):
Thorazine
THERAPEUTIC CLASS:
Antipsychotic
GENERAL USES:
Psychotic/behavioral
disorders, porphyria,
emesis
DOSAGE FORMS:
Tablets: 10 mg, 25
mg, 50 mg, 100 mg,
200 mg; Sustained
release capsules: 30

CHLORTHALIDONE
klor THAL i done
TRADE NAME(S):
Thalitone, Hygroton
THERAPEUTIC CLASS:
Diuretic
GENERAL USES:
CHF related edema,
hypertension
DOSAGE FORMS:
Tablets: 15 mg, 25
mg, 50 mg, 100 mg

CHLORZOXAZONE

klor ZOKS a zone

TRADE NAME(S):
Paraflex, Parafon Forte DSC, Remular

THERAPEUTIC CLASS:
Skeletal muscle relaxant

GENERAL USES:
Musculoskeletal conditions

DOSAGE FORMS:
Tablets & Capsules: 250 mg, 500 mg

CICLOPIROX

sye kloe PEER oks

TRADE NAME(S):
Loprox, Penlac

THERAPEUTIC CLASS:
Antifungal (topical)

GENERAL USES:
Athlete's foot, jock itch, ringworm, nail infections (topical nail preparation)

DOSAGE FORMS:
Cream & Lotion: 1%; Nail lacquer: 8%

CILOSTAZOL

sil OH sta zol

TRADE NAME(S):
Pletal

THERAPEUTIC CLASS:
Antiplatelet agent

GENERAL USES:
Intermittent claudication

DOSAGE FORMS:
Tablets: 50 mg, 100 mg

CIMETIDINE

sye MET i DEEN

TRADE NAME(S):
Tagamet, Tagamet HB

THERAPEUTIC CLASS:
Gastric acid secretion inhibitor

GENERAL USES:
Duodenal ulcer, GERD, heartburn (OTC)

DOSAGE FORMS:
Tablets: 100 mg, 200 mg, 300 mg, 400 mg, 800 mg; Solution: 300 mg/5 mL; Injection: 300 mg, 600 mg

CINOXACIN

sin OKS a sin

TRADE NAME(S):
Cinobac

THERAPEUTIC CLASS:
Anti-infective

GENERAL USES:
Bacterial infections

DOSAGE FORMS:
Capsules: 250 mg, 500 mg

CIPROFLOXACIN
sip roe FLOKS a sin
TRADE NAME(S):
Cipro
THERAPEUTIC CLASS:
Anti-infective
GENERAL USES:
Bacterial infections
DOSAGE FORMS:
Tablets: 100 mg,
250 mg, 500 mg,
750 mg; Suspension:
250 mg/ 5 mL,
500 mg/5 mL;
Injection: 200 mg,
400 mg

CIPROFLOXACIN (OCULAR)
sip roe FLOKS a sin
TRADE NAME(S):
Ciloxan
THERAPEUTIC CLASS:
Ocular agent (anti-infective)
GENERAL USES:
Ocular infections
DOSAGE FORMS:
Ophthalmic solution &
Ointment: 0.3%

CISPLATIN
SIS pla tin
TRADE NAME(S):
Platinol-AQ

THERAPEUTIC CLASS:
Antineoplastic
GENERAL USES:
Cancer of the bladder,
testes, ovaries
DOSAGE FORMS:
Injection: 50 mg,
100 mg, 200 mg

CITALOPRAM
sye TAL oh pram
TRADE NAME(S):
Celexa
THERAPEUTIC CLASS:
Antidepressant
GENERAL USES:
Depression
DOSAGE FORMS:
Tablets: 20 mg, 40 mg

CLARITHROMYCIN
kla RITH roe mye sin
TRADE NAME(S):
Biaxin
THERAPEUTIC CLASS:
Anti-infective
GENERAL USES:
Bacterial infections
DOSAGE FORMS:
Tablets & Extended
release tablets: 250
mg, 500 mg;
Suspension: 125 mg/
5 mL, 250 mg/5 mL

CLINDAMYCIN

klin da MYE sin

TRADE NAME(S):
Cleocin

THERAPEUTIC CLASS:
Anti-infective

GENERAL USES:
Bacterial infections

DOSAGE FORMS:
Capsules: 75 mg, 150 mg, 300 mg; Solution: 75 mg/5 mL; Injection: 300 mg, 600 mg, 900 mg

CLINDAMYCIN (TOPICAL)

klin da MYE sin

TRADE NAME(S):
Cleocin T, Clinda-Derm

THERAPEUTIC CLASS:
Anti-infective (topical)

GENERAL USES:
Acne

DOSAGE FORMS:
Gel, Lotion & Topical Solution: 10 mg/mL

CLINDAMYCIN (VAGINAL)

klin da MYE sin

TRADE NAME(S):
Cleocin

THERAPEUTIC CLASS:
Vaginal anti-infective

GENERAL USES:
Vaginal bacterial infections

DOSAGE FORMS:
Cream: 2%

CLOBETASOL

kloe BAY ta sol

TRADE NAME(S):
Temovate

THERAPEUTIC CLASS:
Corticosteroid (topical)

GENERAL USES:
Various skin conditions

DOSAGE FORMS:
Ointment, Cream & Gel: 0.05%

CLOMIPRAMINE

kloe MI pra meen

TRADE NAME(S):
Anafranil

THERAPEUTIC CLASS:
Antidepressant

GENERAL USES:
Obsessive-compulsive disorder

DOSAGE FORMS:
Capsules: 25 mg, 50 mg, 75 mg

CLONAZEPAM

kloe NA ze pam

TRADE NAME(S):
Klonopin

THERAPEUTIC CLASS:
Anticonvulsant

GENERAL USES:
Seizures

DOSAGE FORMS:
Tablets: 0.5 mg, 1 mg, 2 mg

CLONIDINE

KLON i deen

TRADE NAME(S):
Catapres, Catapres TTS

THERAPEUTIC CLASS:
Antihypertensive

GENERAL USES:
Hypertension

DOSAGE FORMS:
Tablets: 0.1 mg, 0.2 mg, 0.3 mg; Transdermal patch (content): 2.5 mg, 5 mg, 7.5 mg

CLONIDINE/ CHLORTHALIDONE

KLON i deen/klor THAL i done

TRADE NAME(S):
Combipres

THERAPEUTIC CLASS:
Antihypertensive/ diuretic

GENERAL USES:
Hypertension

DOSAGE FORMS:
Tablets: 0.1 mg/15 mg, 0.2 mg/15 mg, 0.3 mg/15 mg

CLOPIDOGREL

kloh PID oh grel

TRADE NAME(S):
Plavix

THERAPEUTIC CLASS:
Antiplatelet agent

GENERAL USES:
Reduce stroke, myocardial infarction risk

DOSAGE FORMS:
Tablets: 75 mg

CLORAZEPATE

klor AZ e pate

TRADE NAME(S):
Tranxene, Gen-Xene

THERAPEUTIC CLASS:
Antianxiety agent, anti-convulsant

GENERAL USES:
Anxiety, panic disorder, seizures

DOSAGE FORMS:
Capsules or Tablets: 3.75 mg, 7.5 mg,

15 mg; Single dose
tablets: 11.25 mg,
22.5 mg

CLOTRIMAZOLE (ORAL)
kloe TRIM a zole
Trade name(s):
Mycelex
Therapeutic Class:
Antifungal
General Uses:
Oral fungal infection
(candidiasis)
Dosage Forms:
Troches: 10 mg

CLOTRIMAZOLE (TOPICAL)
kloe TRIM a zole
Trade name(s):
Lotrimin, Mycelex
Therapeutic Class:
Antifungal (topical)
General Uses:
Athlete's foot, jock
itch, ringworm, tinea
versicolor, candidiasis
Dosage Forms:
Cream, Solution &
Lotion: 1%

CLOXACILLIN
kloks a SIL in
Trade name(s):
Cloxapen
Therapeutic Class:
Anti-infective
General Uses:
Bacterial infections
Dosage Forms:
Capsules: 250 mg,
500 mg; Solution:
125 mg/5 mL

CLOZAPINE
KLOE za peen
Trade name(s):
Clozaril
Therapeutic Class:
Antipsychotic
General Uses:
Psychotic disorders
Dosage Forms:
Tablets: 25 mg,
100 mg

CODEINE SULFATE
KOE deen
Trade name(s):
Codeine
Therapeutic Class:
Analgesic (narcotic)
General Uses:
Pain, cough
Dosage Forms:
Tablets: 15 mg, 30

mg, 60 mg; Soluble
tablets: 30 mg, 60 mg

COLCHICINE
KOL chi seen
Trade name(s):
Colchicine
Therapeutic Class:
Gout agent
General Uses:
Gout
Dosage Forms:
Tablets: 0.5 mg, 0.6 mg

COLESEVELAM
koh le SEV a lam
Trade name(s):
Welchol
Therapeutic Class:
Antilipemic
General Uses:
Hyperlipidemia
Dosage Forms:
Tablets: 625 mg

CROMOLYN (INHALED)
KROE moe lin
Trade name(s):
Intal
Therapeutic Class:
Respiratory inhalant
General Uses:
Asthma, bron-

chospasm
Dosage Forms:
Aerosol spray: 800
mcg/spray; Nebulizer
solution: 20 mg/2 mL

CROMOLYN (OCULAR)
KROE moe lin
Trade name(s):
Crolom
Therapeutic Class:
Ocular agent
General Uses:
Conjunctivitis
Dosage Forms:
Ophthalmic solution:
4%

CROMOLYN (ORAL)
KROE moe lin
Trade name(s):
Gastrocrom
Therapeutic Class:
Mast cell stabilizer
General Uses:
Mastocytosis
Dosage Forms:
Oral concentrate:
100 mg/5 mL

CROTAMITON
kroe TAM i tonn
Trade name(s):

Eurax

THERAPEUTIC CLASS:
Scabicide (topical)
GENERAL USES:
Scabies, pruritis
DOSAGE FORMS:
Cream & Lotion: 10%

CYCLOBENZAPRINE
sye kloe BEN za preen
TRADE NAME(S):
Flexeril
THERAPEUTIC CLASS:
Skeletal muscle relaxant
GENERAL USES:
Musculoskeletal conditions
DOSAGE FORMS:
Tablets: 10 mg

CYCLOPHOS-PHAMIDE
sye kloe FOS fa mide
TRADE NAME(S):
Cytoxan
THERAPEUTIC CLASS:
Antineoplastic
GENERAL USES:
Various lymphomas and leukemias
DOSAGE FORMS:
Tablets: 25 mg, 50 mg; Injection: 100 mg, 200 mg, 500 mg, 1 g, 2 g

CYCLOSERINE
sye kloe SER een
TRADE NAME(S):
Seromycin
THERAPEUTIC CLASS:
Antituberculosis agent
GENERAL USES:
Tuberculosis
DOSAGE FORMS:
Capsules: 250 mg

CYCLOSPORINE
SYE kloe spor een
TRADE NAME(S):
Sandimmune, Neoral, SangCya
THERAPEUTIC CLASS:
Immunosuppressant
GENERAL USES:
Rheumatoid arthritis, psoriasis, prevent organ rejection
DOSAGE FORMS:
Capsules: 25 mg, 50 mg, 100 mg; Solution: 100 mg/mL; Injection: 250 mg

CYPROHEPTADINE
si proe HEP ta deen
TRADE NAME(S):
Periactin
THERAPEUTIC CLASS:
Antihistamine

GENERAL USES:
Allergies
DOSAGE FORMS:
Tablets: 4 mg; Syrup:
2 mg/5 mL

DALTEPARIN SODIUM
dal TE pa rin
TRADE NAME(S):
Fragmin
THERAPEUTIC CLASS:
Anticoagulant (LMWH)
GENERAL USES:
Prevention of blood
clots
DOSAGE FORMS:
Injection: 2500 IU,
5000 IU, 95,000 IU

DANAPAROID SODIUM
da NAP a roid
TRADE NAME(S):
Orgaran
THERAPEUTIC CLASS:
Anticoagulant
GENERAL USES:
Prevention of blood
clots
DOSAGE FORMS:
Injection: 750 anti-Xa
units

DANTROLENE
DAN troe leen
TRADE NAME(S):
Dantrium
THERAPEUTIC CLASS:
Skeletal muscle relax-
ant
GENERAL USES:
Spasticity
DOSAGE FORMS:
Capsules: 25 mg, 50
mg, 100 mg; Injection:
20 mg

DARBEPOETIN ALFA
dar be POE e tin AL fa
TRADE NAME(S):
Aranesp
THERAPEUTIC CLASS:
Hematological agent
GENERAL USES:
Anemia
DOSAGE FORMS:
Injection: 0.025 mg,
0.04 mg, 0.06 mg, 0.1
mg, 0.2 mg

DELAVIRDINE
de la VIR deen
TRADE NAME(S):
Rescriptor
THERAPEUTIC CLASS:
Antiviral
GENERAL USES:
HIV infection

DOSAGE FORMS:
Tablets: 100 mg;
Capsules: 200 mg

DEMECARIUM
dem e KARE ee um
TRADE NAME(S):
Humorsol
THERAPEUTIC CLASS:
Ocular agent
GENERAL USES:
Glaucoma
DOSAGE FORMS:
Ophthalmic solution:
0.125%, 0.25%

DEMECLOCYCLINE
dem e kloe SYE kleen
TRADE NAME(S):
Declomycin
THERAPEUTIC CLASS:
Anti-infective
GENERAL USES:
Bacterial infections
DOSAGE FORMS:
Tablets: 150 mg,
300 mg

DESIPRAMINE
des IP ra meen
TRADE NAME(S):
Norpramin
THERAPEUTIC CLASS:
Antidepressant

GENERAL USES:
Depression
DOSAGE FORMS:
Tablets: 10 mg, 25
mg, 50 mg, 75 mg,
100 mg, 150 mg

DESLORATADINE
des lor AT a deen
TRADE NAME(S):
Clarinex, Clarinex
Redi-tabs
THERAPEUTIC CLASS:
Antihistamine
GENERAL USES:
Allergic rhinitis
DOSAGE FORMS:
Tablets: 5 mg; Orally
disintegrating tablets:
5 mg

DESONIDE
DES oh nide
TRADE NAME(S):
DesOwen, Tridesilon
THERAPEUTIC CLASS:
Corticosteroid (topical)
GENERAL USES:
Various skin conditions
DOSAGE FORMS:
Ointment, Cream &
Lotion: 0.05%

DEXAMETHASONE (OCULAR)

deks a METH a sone

TRADE NAME(S):
AK-Dex, Maxidex

THERAPEUTIC CLASS:
Ocular agent (steroid)

GENERAL USES:
Ocular inflammation

DOSAGE FORMS:
Ophthalmic solution, Suspension, Ointment: 0.1%

DEXAMETHASONE (ORAL)

deks a METH a sone

TRADE NAME(S):
Decadron, Dexone, Hexadrol

THERAPEUTIC CLASS:
Glucocorticoid

GENERAL USES:
Endocrine, skin, blood disorders

DOSAGE FORMS:
Tablets: 0.25 mg, 0.5 mg, 0.75 mg, 1 mg, 1.5 mg, 2 mg, 4 mg, 6 mg; Elixir & Solution: 0.5 mg/5 mL; Concentrated solution: 1 mg/1 mL

DEXAMETHASONE ACETATE

deks a METH a sone

TRADE NAME(S):
Dalalone LA, Decadron LA

THERAPEUTIC CLASS:
Glucocorticoid

GENERAL USES:
Endocrine, skin, blood disorders

DOSAGE FORMS:
Injection: 8 mg, 16 mg, 40 mg, 80 mg

DEXAMETHASONE SODIUM PHOSPHATE

deks a METH a sone

TRADE NAME(S):
Dalalone, Decadron Phosphate, Dexasone

THERAPEUTIC CLASS:
Glucocorticoid

GENERAL USES:
Endocrine, skin, blood disorders

DOSAGE FORMS:
Injection: 4 mg, 10 mg, 20 mg, 40 mg, 100 mg, 120 mg, 240 mg

DEXMETHYLPHENIDATE

dex meth il FEN i date

TRADE NAME(S):
Focalin

THERAPEUTIC CLASS:
CNS stimulant

GENERAL USES:
Attention deficit hyper-
activity disorder

DOSAGE FORMS:
Tablets: 2.5 mg, 5 mg,
10 mg

DEXTROAMPHETAMINE SULFATE

deks troe am FET a meen

TRADE NAME(S):
Dexedrine

THERAPEUTIC CLASS:
Amphetamine

GENERAL USES:
Obesity

DOSAGE FORMS:
Tablets: 5 mg, 10 mg;
Sustained release cap-
sules: 5 mg, 10 mg,
15 mg; Elixir: 5 mg/5
mL

DEXTROAMPHETAMINE/ AMPHETAMINE

deks troe am FET a
meen/am FET a meen

TRADE NAME(S):
Adderall, Adderall XR

THERAPEUTIC CLASS:
Amphetamine

GENERAL USES:
Attention deficit disor-
der

DOSAGE FORMS:
Tablets: 5 mg, 10 mg,
20 mg, 30 mg;
Extended release cap-
sules: 10 mg, 20 mg,
30 mg

DIAZEPAM

dye AZ e pam

TRADE NAME(S):
Valium

THERAPEUTIC CLASS:
Antianxiety agent, anti-
convulsant, muscle
relaxant

GENERAL USES:
Anxiety, alcohol with-
drawal, seizures, mus-
cle relaxant

DOSAGE FORMS:
Tablets: 2 mg, 5 mg,
10 mg; Solution: 5
mg/5 mL, 5 mg/mL;
Injection: 10 mg, 50
mg

DICLOFENAC (OCULAR)

dye KLOE fen ak

TRADE NAME(S):
Voltaren

THERAPEUTIC CLASS:
Ocular agent

GENERAL USES:
Postoperative ocular inflammation

DOSAGE FORMS:
Ophthalmic solution: 0.1%

DICLOFENAC (ORAL)

dye KLOE fen ak

TRADE NAME(S):
Cataflam, Voltaren, Voltaren-XR

THERAPEUTIC CLASS:
Anti-inflammatory/ analgesic

GENERAL USES:
Osteoarthritis, rheumatoid arthritis, pain

DOSAGE FORMS:
Tablets & Delayed release tablets: 25 mg, 50 mg, 75 mg; Extended release tablets: 100 mg

DICLOFENAC/ MISOPROSTOL

dye KLOE fen ak/mye soe PROST ole

TRADE NAME(S):
Arthrotec

THERAPEUTIC CLASS:
Analgesic/GI protectant

GENERAL USES:
Arthritis

DOSAGE FORMS:
Tablets: 50 mg/200 mcg, 75 mg/200 mcg

DICLOXACILLIN

dye kloks a SIL in

TRADE NAME(S):
Dynapen, Dycill, Pathocil

THERAPEUTIC CLASS:
Anti-infective

GENERAL USES:
Bacterial infections

DOSAGE FORMS:
Capsules: 125 mg, 250 mg, 500 mg; Suspension: 62.5 mg/5 mL

DICYCLOMINE

dye SYE kloe meen

TRADE NAME(S):
Bentyl, Byclomine, Di-Spaz

THERAPEUTIC CLASS:
Gastrointestinal anti-spasmodic

GENERAL USES:
Irritable bowel syndrome

DOSAGE FORMS:
Capsules: 10 mg, 20 mg; Tablets: 20 mg; Syrup: 10 mg/5 mL

DIDANOSINE (ddI)
dye DAN oh seen

TRADE NAME(S):
Videx, Videx EC

THERAPEUTIC CLASS:
Antiviral

GENERAL USES:
HIV infection

DOSAGE FORMS:
Chewable tablets: 25 mg, 50 mg, 100 mg, 150 mg, 200 mg; Powder: 100 mg, 167 mg, 250 mg, 375 mg, 2 g, 4 g; Delayed release capsules: 125 mg, 200 mg, 250 mg, 400 mg

DIFLUNISAL
dye FLOO ni sal

TRADE NAME(S):
Dolobid

THERAPEUTIC CLASS:
Anti-inflammatory/analgesic

GENERAL USES:
Pain, osteoarthritis, rheumatoid arthritis

DOSAGE FORMS:
Tablets: 250 mg, 500 mg

DIGOXIN
di JOKS in

TRADE NAME(S):
Lanoxicaps, Lanoxin

THERAPEUTIC CLASS:
Cardiac agent

GENERAL USES:
Congestive heart failure, atrial fibrillation

DOSAGE FORMS:
Capsules: 0.05 mg, 0.1 mg, 0.2 mg; Tablets: 0.125 mg, 0.25 mg, 0.5 mg; Elixir: 0.05 mg/mL; Injection: 0.1 mg, 0.5 mg

DIHYDROERGOTAMINE
dye hye droe er GOT a meen

TRADE NAME(S):
Migranal

THERAPEUTIC CLASS:
Anti-migraine agent

GENERAL USES:
  Migraines
DOSAGE FORMS:
  Nasal spray: 4 mg/mL

DILTIAZEM
dil TYE a zem
TRADE NAME(S):
  Cardizem CD,
  Cardizem SR, Dilacor
  XR, Tiazac
THERAPEUTIC CLASS:
  Antihypertensive,
  antianginal
GENERAL USES:
  Hypertension, angina
DOSAGE FORMS:
  Tablets: 30 mg, 60
  mg, 90 mg, 120 mg;
  Extended release
  tablets: 120 mg, 180
  mg, 240 mg;
  Sustained release cap-
  sules: 60 mg, 90 mg,
  120 mg, 180 mg, 300
  mg; Injection: 25 mg,
  50 mg

DILTIAZEM/
ENALAPRIL
dil TYE a zem/e NAL a
pril
TRADE NAME(S):
  Teczem

THERAPEUTIC CLASS:
  Antihypertensive
GENERAL USES:
  Hypertension
DOSAGE FORMS:
  Extended release
  tablets: 180 mg/5 mg

DIMENHYDRINATE
die men HIGH drih nate
TRADE NAME(S):
  Hydrate, Dramanate
THERAPEUTIC CLASS:
  Antiemetic/antivertigo
  agent
GENERAL USES:
  Motion sickness
DOSAGE FORMS:
  Tablets: 50 mg

DIPHENHYDRAMINE
dye fen HYE dra meen
TRADE NAME(S):
  Benadryl, Tusstat,
  Hyrexin-50
THERAPEUTIC CLASS:
  Antihistamine,
  antiemetic
GENERAL USES:
  Pruritus, allergies,
  sleep aid, cough aid
DOSAGE FORMS:
  Tablets & Capsules: 25
  mg, 50 mg; Chewable
  tablets: 12.5 mg;

Liquid, Solution, Elixir, & Syrup: 12.5 mg/5 mL; Cream: 1%, 2%

DIPIVEFRIN
dye PI ve frin
TRADE NAME(S):
Propine, AKPro
THERAPEUTIC CLASS:
Ocular agent
GENERAL USES:
Glaucoma
DOSAGE FORMS:
Ophthalmic solution: 0.1%

DIPYRIDAMOLE
dye peer ID a mole
TRADE NAME(S):
Persantine
THERAPEUTIC CLASS:
Antiplatelet agent
GENERAL USES:
Preventive therapy for blood clots
DOSAGE FORMS:
Tablets: 25 mg, 50 mg, 75 mg

DIRITHROMYCIN
dye RITH roe mye sin
TRADE NAME(S):
Dynabac

THERAPEUTIC CLASS:
Anti-infective
GENERAL USES:
Bacterial infections
DOSAGE FORMS:
Tablets: 250 mg

DISOPYRAMIDE
dye soe PEER a mide
TRADE NAME(S):
Norpace, Norpace CR
THERAPEUTIC CLASS:
Antiarrhythmic
GENERAL USES:
Ventricular arrhythmias
DOSAGE FORMS:
Capsules and Extended release capsules: 100 mg, 150 mg

DISULFIRAM
dye SUL fi ram
TRADE NAME(S):
Antabuse
THERAPEUTIC CLASS:
Antialcoholic
GENERAL USES:
Alcohol abstinence
DOSAGE FORMS:
Tablets: 250 mg, 500 mg

DOBUTAMINE

doe BYOO ta meen

TRADE NAME(S):
Dobutrex

THERAPEUTIC CLASS:
Cardiac agent

GENERAL USES:
Increases cardiac contractility

DOSAGE FORMS:
Injection: 250 mg

DOCOSANOL

doe KOE san ole

TRADE NAME(S):
Abreva

THERAPEUTIC CLASS:
Antiviral

GENERAL USES:
Treatment of fever blisters, cold sores

DOSAGE FORMS:
Cream: 10%

DOFETILIDE

doe FET il ide

TRADE NAME(S):
Tikosyn

THERAPEUTIC CLASS:
Antiarrhythmic

GENERAL USES:
Atrial fibrillation/flutter

DOSAGE FORMS:
Capsules: 125 mcg, 250 mcg, 500 mcg

DOLASETRON

dol A se tron

TRADE NAME(S):
Anzemet

THERAPEUTIC CLASS:
Antiemetic

GENERAL USES:
Surgical or chemotherapy nausea/vomiting

DOSAGE FORMS:
Tablets: 50 mg, 100 mg; Injection: 12.5 mg, 100 mg

DONEPEZIL

doh NEP e zil

TRADE NAME(S):
Aricept

THERAPEUTIC CLASS:
Alzheimer's agent

GENERAL USES:
Alzheimer's disease

DOSAGE FORMS:
Tablets: 5 mg, 10 mg

DOPAMINE

DOE pa meen

TRADE NAME(S):
Intropin

THERAPEUTIC CLASS:
Cardiac agent

GENERAL USES:
Increases cardiac output

DOSAGE FORMS:
Injection: 200 mg, 400 mg, 800 mg, 1.6 g

DORZOLAMIDE
dor ZOLE a mide
TRADE NAME(S):
Trusopt
THERAPEUTIC CLASS:
Ocular agent
GENERAL USES:
Glaucoma/ocular hypertension
DOSAGE FORMS:
Ophthalmic solution: 2%

DORZOLAMIDE/ TIMOLOL
dor ZOLE a mide/TYE moe lole
TRADE NAME(S):
Cosopt
THERAPEUTIC CLASS:
Ocular agent
GENERAL USES:
Glaucoma/ocular hypertension
DOSAGE FORMS:
Ophthalmic solution: 2%/0.5%

DOXAZOSIN
doks AY zoe sin

TRADE NAME(S):
Cardura
THERAPEUTIC CLASS:
Antihypertensive, BPH agent
GENERAL USES:
Hypertension, benign prostatic hypertrophy
DOSAGE FORMS:
Tablets: 1 mg, 2 mg, 4 mg, 8 mg

DOXEPIN (ORAL)
DOKS e pin
TRADE NAME(S):
Sinequan
THERAPEUTIC CLASS:
Antidepressant
GENERAL USES:
Depression
DOSAGE FORMS:
Capsules: 10 mg, 25 mg, 50 mg, 75 mg, 100 mg, 150 mg; Solution: 10 mg/mL

DOXEPIN (TOPICAL)
DOKS e pin
TRADE NAME(S):
Zonalon
THERAPEUTIC CLASS:
Antipruritic (topical)
GENERAL USES:
Pruritus

DOSAGE FORMS:
  Cream: 5%

DOXYCYCLINE
doks i SYE kleen
TRADE NAME(S):
  Vibramycin, Vibra-Tabs, Doxy, Doxychel
THERAPEUTIC CLASS:
  Anti-infective
GENERAL USES:
  Bacterial infections
DOSAGE FORMS:
  Capsules: 20 mg, 50 mg, 100 mg; Tablets: 50 mg, 100 mg; Suspension: 25 mg/5 mL; Syrup: 50 mg/5 mL

DOXYCYCLINE
doks i SYE kleen
TRADE NAME(S):
  Atridox
THERAPEUTIC CLASS:
  Anti-infective
GENERAL USES:
  Periodontitis
DOSAGE FORMS:
  Oral gel: 10%

DRONABINOL
droe NAB i nol
TRADE NAME(S):
  Marinol
THERAPEUTIC CLASS:
  Antiemetic
GENERAL USES:
  Chemotherapy nausea/vomiting, appetite stimulant
DOSAGE FORMS:
  Capsules: 2.5 mg, 5 mg, 10 mg

DROTRECOGIN ALFA
dro TRE coe jin AL fa
TRADE NAME(S):
  Xigris
THERAPEUTIC CLASS:
  Biological
GENERAL USES:
  Sepsis
DOSAGE FORMS:
  Injection: 5 mg, 20 mg

ECONAZOLE
e KONE a zole
TRADE NAME(S):
  Spectazole
THERAPEUTIC CLASS:
  Antifungal (topical)
GENERAL USES:
  Athlete's foot, jock itch, ringworm
DOSAGE FORMS:
  Cream: 1%

EFAVIRENZ
e FAV e renz
TRADE NAME(S):
  Sustiva
THERAPEUTIC CLASS:
  Antiviral
GENERAL USES:
  HIV infection
DOSAGE FORMS:
  Capsules: 50 mg,
  100 mg, 200 mg

EMEDASTINE
em e DAS teen
TRADE NAME(S):
  Emadine
THERAPEUTIC CLASS:
  Ocular agent
GENERAL USES:
  Allergic conjunctivitis
DOSAGE FORMS:
  Ophthalmic solution:
  0.05%

ENALAPRIL
e NAL a pril
TRADE NAME(S):
  Vasotec, Vasotec IV
THERAPEUTIC CLASS:
  Antihypertensive,
  cardiac agent
GENERAL USES:
  Hypertension, heart
  failure, left ventricular
  dysfunction

DOSAGE FORMS:
  Tablets: 2.5 mg,
  5 mg, 10 mg, 20 mg;
  Injection: 1.25 mg,
  2.5 mg (enalaprilat)

ENALAPRIL/ FELODIPINE
e NAL a pril/fe LOE di
peen
TRADE NAME(S):
  Lexxel
THERAPEUTIC CLASS:
  Antihypertensive
GENERAL USES:
  Hypertension
DOSAGE FORMS:
  Extended release
  tablets: 5 mg/2.5 mg,
  5 mg/5 mg

ENALAPRIL/HCTZ
e NAL a pril/hye droe
klor oh THYE a zide
TRADE NAME(S):
  Vaseretic
THERAPEUTIC CLASS:
  Antihypertensive/
  diuretic
GENERAL USES:
  Hypertension
DOSAGE FORMS:
  Tablets: 5 mg/12.5
  mg, 10 mg/25 mg

ENOXACIN
en OX a sin
TRADE NAME(S):
  Penetrex
THERAPEUTIC CLASS:
  Anti-infective
GENERAL USES:
  Bacterial infections
DOSAGE FORMS:
  Tablets: 200 mg,
  400 mg

ENOXAPARIN SODIUM
ee noks a PA rin
TRADE NAME(S):
  Lovenox
THERAPEUTIC CLASS:
  Anticoagulant (LMWH)
GENERAL USES:
  Prevention of blood
  clots
DOSAGE FORMS:
  Injection: 30 mg,
  40 mg, 60 mg, 80 mg,
  90 mg, 100 mg,
  120 mg, 150 mg

ENTACAPONE
en TA ka pone
TRADE NAME(S):
  Comtan
THERAPEUTIC CLASS:
  Antiparkinson agent

GENERAL USES:
  Parkinson's disease
DOSAGE FORMS:
  Tablets: 200 mg

EPINEPHRINE
ep i NEF rin
TRADE NAME(S):
  Epifrin, Glaucon
THERAPEUTIC CLASS:
  Ocular agent
GENERAL USES:
  Glaucoma
DOSAGE FORMS:
  Ophthalmic solution:
  0.1%, 0.5%, 1%, 2%

EPLERENONE
e PLER en one
TRADE NAME(S):
  Inspra
THERAPEUTIC CLASS:
  Antihypertensive
GENERAL USES:
  Hypertension
DOSAGE FORMS:
  Tablets: 25 mg, 50
  mg, 100 mg

EPOETIN ALFA
e POE e tin AL fa
TRADE NAME(S):
  Epogen, Procrit

THERAPEUTIC CLASS:
Hematological agent
GENERAL USES:
Anemia with chronic renal failure, cancer or HIV infection
DOSAGE FORMS:
Injection: 2000 units, 3000 units, 4000 units, 10,000 units, 20,000 units

ERGOTAMINE TARTRATE
er GOT a meen
TRADE NAME(S):
Ergomar
THERAPEUTIC CLASS:
Antimigraine agent
GENERAL USES:
Migraines
DOSAGE FORMS:
Sublingual tablets: 2 mg

ERTAPENEM
er ta PEN em
TRADE NAME(S):
Invanz
THERAPEUTIC CLASS:
Anti-infective
GENERAL USES:
Bacterial infections
DOSAGE FORMS:
Injection: 1 g

ERYTHROMYCIN (BASE)
er ith roe MYE sin
TRADE NAME(S):
E-Mycin, E-Base, PCE, Ery-Tab, Eryc
THERAPEUTIC CLASS:
Anti-infective
GENERAL USES:
Bacterial infections
DOSAGE FORMS:
Tablets: 250 mg, 333 mg, 500 mg; Delayed release capsules: 250 mg

ERYTHROMYCIN (OCULAR)
er ith roe MYE sin
TRADE NAME(S):
Ilotycin
THERAPEUTIC CLASS:
Ocular agent (anti-infective)
GENERAL USES:
Ocular infections
DOSAGE FORMS:
Ophthalmic ointment: 5%

ERYTHROMYCIN (TOPICAL)

er ith roe MYE sin

TRADE NAME(S):
Akne-mycin, Emgel, Erygel

THERAPEUTIC CLASS:
Anti-infective (topical)

GENERAL USES:
Acne

DOSAGE FORMS:
Ointment & Gel: 2%; Solution: 1.5%, 2%

ERYTHROMYCIN ESTOLATE

er ith roe MYE sin

TRADE NAME(S):
Ilosone

THERAPEUTIC CLASS:
Anti-infective

GENERAL USES:
Bacterial infections

DOSAGE FORMS:
Tablets: 500 mg; Capsules: 250 mg; Suspension: 125 mg/ 5 mL, 250 mg/5 mL

ERYTHROMYCIN ETHYLSUCCINATE

er ith roe MYE sin

TRADE NAME(S):
EryPed, EES

THERAPEUTIC CLASS:
Anti-infective

GENERAL USES:
Bacterial infections

DOSAGE FORMS:
Tablets: 400 mg; Chewable tablets: 200 mg; Suspension: 200 mg/5 mL, 400 mg/5 mL, 100 mg/2.5 mL

ERYTHROMYCIN LACTOBIONATE

er ith roe MYE sin

TRADE NAME(S):
Erythrocin

THERAPEUTIC CLASS:
Anti-infective

GENERAL USES:
Bacterial infections

DOSAGE FORMS:
Injection: 500 mg, 1 g

ERYTHROMYCIN STEARATE

er ith roe MYE sin

TRADE NAME(S):
Erythrocin

THERAPEUTIC CLASS:
Anti-infective

GENERAL USES:
Bacterial infections

DOSAGE FORMS:
Tablets: 250 mg, 500 mg

ERYTHROMYCIN/ BENZOYL PEROXIDE

er ith roe MYE sin/BEN zoe il per OKS ide

TRADE NAME(S):
Benzamycin

THERAPEUTIC CLASS:
Anti-infective (topical)

GENERAL USES:
Acne

DOSAGE FORMS:
Gel: 30 mg/50 mg per g

ESCITALOPRAM

es sye TAL oh pram

TRADE NAME(S):
Lexapro

THERAPEUTIC CLASS:
Antidepressant

GENERAL USES:
Depression

DOSAGE FORMS:
Tablets: 5 mg, 10 mg, 20 mg

ESOMEPRAZOLE

es oh ME pray zol

TRADE NAME(S):
Nexium

THERAPEUTIC CLASS:
Gastric acid secretion inhibitor

GENERAL USES:
GERD, erosive esophagitis

DOSAGE FORMS:
Capsules: 20 mg, 40 mg

ESTAZOLAM

es TA zoe lam

TRADE NAME(S):
ProSom

THERAPEUTIC CLASS:
Sedative/hypnotic

GENERAL USES:
Insomnia

DOSAGE FORMS:
Tablets: 1 mg, 2 mg

ESTRADIOL (TRANSDERMAL)

es tra DYE ole

TRADE NAME(S):
FemPatch, Vivelle, Alora, Estraderm, Climara

THERAPEUTIC CLASS:
Hormone (estrogen)

GENERAL USES:
Estrogen replacement

DOSAGE FORMS:
Transdermal patch (release rate/24 hr): 0.025 mg, 0.0375 mg, 0.05 mg, 0.075 mg, 0.1 mg

ESTRADIOL/ NORETHINDRONE

es tra DYE ole/nor eth IN drone

TRADE NAME(S):
Activella

THERAPEUTIC CLASS:
Hormone (estrogen/progestin)

GENERAL USES:
Estrogen replacement

DOSAGE FORMS:
Tablets: 1 mg/0.5 mg

ESTROGENS, CONJUGATED

ES troe jenz, KON joo gate ed

TRADE NAME(S):
Premarin, Premarin IV

THERAPEUTIC CLASS:
Hormone (estrogen)

GENERAL USES:
Estrogen replacement

DOSAGE FORMS:
Tablets: 0.3 mg, 0.625 mg, 0.9 mg, 1.25 mg, 2.5 mg; Injection: 25 mg

ESTROGENS, ESTERIFIED

ES troe jenz, es TER i fied

TRADE NAME(S):
Estratab, Menest

THERAPEUTIC CLASS:
Hormone (estrogen)

GENERAL USES:
Estrogen replacement

DOSAGE FORMS:
Tablets: 0.3 mg, 0.625 mg, 1.25 mg, 2.5 mg

ESTROGENS/ MEDROXY-PROGESTERONE

ES troe jenz/me DROKS ee proe JES te rone

TRADE NAME(S):
Prempro, Premphase

THERAPEUTIC CLASS:
Hormone (estrogen/progestin)

GENERAL USES:
Estrogen replacement

DOSAGE FORMS:
Tablets: 0.625 mg/5 mg, 0.625 mg/2.5 mg

ESTROPIPATE

ES troe pih pate

TRADE NAME(S):
Ogen, Ortho-Est

THERAPEUTIC CLASS:
Hormone (estrogen)

GENERAL USES:
Estrogen replacement

DOSAGE FORMS:
Tablets: 0.625 mg,

1.25 mg, 2.5 mg,
5 mg; Vaginal cream:
0.15%

ETHACRYNIC ACID
eth a KRIN ik AS id
TRADE NAME(S):
Edecrin
THERAPEUTIC CLASS:
Diuretic
GENERAL USES:
CHF related edema,
hypertension
DOSAGE FORMS:
Tablets: 25 mg, 50 mg

ETHAMBUTOL
e THAM byoo tole
TRADE NAME(S):
Myambutol
THERAPEUTIC CLASS:
Antituberculosis agent
GENERAL USES:
Tuberculosis
DOSAGE FORMS:
Tablets: 100 mg,
400 mg

ETHINYL ESTRADIOL
ETH in il es tra DYE ole
TRADE NAME(S):
Estinyl
THERAPEUTIC CLASS:
Hormone (estrogen)

GENERAL USES:
Estrogen replacement
DOSAGE FORMS:
Tablets: 0.02 mg, 0.05
mg, 0.25 mg, 0.5 mg

ETHINYL ESTRADIOL/
DESOGESTREL
ETH in il es tra DYE
ole/des oh JES trel
TRADE NAME(S):
Desogen, Ortho-Cept
THERAPEUTIC CLASS:
Contraceptive
(monophasic)
GENERAL USES:
Contraception
DOSAGE FORMS:
Tablets: 30 mcg/0.15
mg

ETHINYL ESTRADIOL/
DESOGESTREL
ETH in il es tra DYE ole/des
oh JES trel
TRADE NAME(S):
Mircette
THERAPEUTIC CLASS:
Contraceptive (biphasic)
GENERAL USES:
Contraception
DOSAGE FORMS:
Tablets: Phase 1: 20
mcg/0.15 mg; Phase
2: 10 mcg (EE)

ETHINYL ESTRADIOL/ DROSPIRENONE
ETH in il es tra DYE ole/droh SPYE re none
TRADE NAME(S):
Yasmin
THERAPEUTIC CLASS:
Contraceptive (monophasic)
GENERAL USES:
Contraception
DOSAGE FORMS:
Tablets: 0.03 mg/3 mg

ETHINYL ESTRADIOL/ ETHYNODIOL
ETH in il es tra DYE ole/e thye noe DYE ole
TRADE NAME(S):
Demulen 1/50, Zovia 1/50E
THERAPEUTIC CLASS:
Contraceptive (monophasic)
GENERAL USES:
Contraception
DOSAGE FORMS:
Tablets: 50 mcg/1 mg

ETHINYL ESTRADIOL/ ETHYNODIOL
ETH in il es tra DYE ole/e thye noe DYE ole
TRADE NAME(S):
Demulen 1/35, Zovia 1/35E
THERAPEUTIC CLASS:
Contraceptive (monophasic)
GENERAL USES:
Contraception
DOSAGE FORMS:
Tablets: 35 mcg/1 mg

ETHINYL ESTRADIOL/ ETONOGESTREL
ETH in il es tra DYE ole/et oh noe JES trel
TRADE NAME(S):
NuvaRing
THERAPEUTIC CLASS:
Contraceptive
GENERAL USES:
Contraception
DOSAGE FORMS:
Vaginal ring (release rate/24 hrs): 15 mcg/120 mcg

ETHINYL ESTRADIOL/ LEVONORGESTREL
ETH in il es tra DYE ole/LEE voe nor jes trel
TRADE NAME(S):
Preven
THERAPEUTIC CLASS:
Contraceptive (emergency)

GENERAL USES:
Emergency contraception

DOSAGE FORMS:
Tablets: 50 mcg/0.25 mg

ETHINYL ESTRADIOL/ LEVONORGESTREL
ETH in il es tra DYE ole/LEE voe nor jes trel
TRADE NAME(S):
Levlen, Levora 0.15/30, Nordette
THERAPEUTIC CLASS:
Contraceptive (monophasic)
GENERAL USES:
Contraception
DOSAGE FORMS:
Tablets: 30 mcg/0.15 mg

ETHINYL ESTRADIOL/ LEVONORGESTREL
ETH in il es tra DYE ole/LEE voe nor jes trel
TRADE NAME(S):
Alesse
THERAPEUTIC CLASS:
Contraceptive (monophasic)
GENERAL USES:
Contraception

DOSAGE FORMS:
Tablets: 20 mcg/0.1 mg

ETHINYL ESTRADIOL/ LEVONORGESTREL
ETH in il es tra DYE ole/LEE voe nor jes trel
TRADE NAME(S):
Levlite
THERAPEUTIC CLASS:
Contraceptive (monophasic)
GENERAL USES:
Contraception
DOSAGE FORMS:
Tablets: 20 mcg/0.1 mg

ETHINYL ESTRADIOL/ LEVONORGESTREL
ETH in il es tra DYE ole/LEE voe nor jes trel
TRADE NAME(S):
Tri-Levlen, Triphasil, Trivora-28
THERAPEUTIC CLASS:
Contraceptive (triphasic)
GENERAL USES:
Contraception
DOSAGE FORMS:
Tablets: Phase 1: 30 mcg/0.05 mg; Phase 2: 40 mcg/0.075 mg; Phase 3: 30 mcg/0.125 mg

ETHINYL ESTRADIOL/ NORELGESTROMIN

ETH in il es tra DYE
ole/nor el JES troe min

TRADE NAME(S):
Ortho Evra

THERAPEUTIC CLASS:
Contraceptive

GENERAL USES:
Contraception

DOSAGE FORMS:
Transdermal patch
(release rate/24 hrs):
20 mcg/150 mcg

ETHINYL ESTRADIOL/ NORETHINDRONE

ETH in il es tra DYE
ole/nor eth IN drone

TRADE NAME(S):
Ovcon-50

THERAPEUTIC CLASS:
Contraceptive
(monophasic)

GENERAL USES:
Contraception

DOSAGE FORMS:
Tablets: 50 mcg/1 mg

ETHINYL ESTRADIOL/ NORETHINDRONE

ETH in il es tra DYE
ole/nor eth IN drone

TRADE NAME(S):
Genora 1/35, Nelova

1/35E, Norethin
1/35E, Norinyl 1+35,
Necon 1/35, Ortho-
Novum 1/35

THERAPEUTIC CLASS:
Contraceptive
(monophasic)

GENERAL USES:
Contraception

DOSAGE FORMS:
Tablets: 35 mcg/1 mg

ETHINYL ESTRADIOL/ NORETHINDRONE

ETH in il es tra DYE
ole/nor eth IN drone

TRADE NAME(S):
Brevicon, Modicon,
Genora 0.5/35, Nelova
0.5/35E, Necon
0.5/35

THERAPEUTIC CLASS:
Contraceptive
(monophasic)

GENERAL USES:
Contraception

DOSAGE FORMS:
Tablets: 35 mcg/0.5 mg

ETHINYL ESTRADIOL/ NORETHINDRONE

ETH in il es tra DYE
ole/nor eth IN drone

TRADE NAME(S):
Ovcon 35

Therapeutic Class:
  Contraceptive
  (monophasic)
General Uses:
  Contraception
Dosage Forms:
  Tablets: 35 mcg/0.4 mg

Dosage Forms:
  Tablets: 20 mcg/1 mg

ETHINYL ESTRADIOL/ NORETHINDRONE
ETH in il es tra DYE
ole/nor eth IN drone
Trade name(s):
  Loestrin 1.5/30
Therapeutic Class:
  Contraceptive
  (monophasic)
General Uses:
  Contraception
Dosage Forms:
  Tablets: 30 mcg/1.5
  mg

ETHINYL ESTRADIOL/ NORETHINDRONE
ETH in il es tra DYE
ole/nor eth IN drone
Trade name(s):
  Loestrin 1/20, Loestrin
  Fe 1/20
Therapeutic Class:
  Contraceptive
  (monophasic)
General Uses:
  Contraception

ETHINYL ESTRADIOL/ NORETHINDRONE
ETH in il es tra DYE
ole/nor eth IN drone
Trade name(s):
  Jenest-28, Nelova
  10/11, Ortho-Novum
  10/11, Necon 10/11
Therapeutic Class:
  Contraceptive (biphasic)
General Uses:
  Contraception
Dosage Forms:
  Tablets: Phase 1: 35
  mcg/0.5 mg; Phase 2:
  35 mcg/1 mg

ETHINYL ESTRADIOL/ NORETHINDRONE
ETH in il es tra DYE
ole/nor eth IN drone
Trade name(s):
  Tri-Norinyl
Therapeutic Class:
  Contraceptive (triphasic)
General Uses:
  Contraception
Dosage Forms:
  Tablets: Phase 1: 35
  mcg/0.5 mg; Phase 2:
  35 mcg/1 mg; Phase

3: 35 mcg/0.5 mg

ETHINYL ESTRADIOL/ NORETHINDRONE

ETH in il es tra DYE
ole/nor eth IN drone

TRADE NAME(S):
Ortho-Novum 7/7/7

THERAPEUTIC CLASS:
Contraceptive (triphasic)

GENERAL USES:
Contraception

DOSAGE FORMS:
Tablets: Phase 1: 35
mcg/0.5 mg; Phase 2:
35 mcg/0.75 mg;
Phase 3: 35 mcg/1 mg

ETHINYL ESTRADIOL/ NORETHINDRONE

ETH in il es tra DYE
ole/nor eth IN drone

TRADE NAME(S):
Estrostep

THERAPEUTIC CLASS:
Contraceptive (triphasic)

GENERAL USES:
Contraception

DOSAGE FORMS:
Tablets: Phase 1: 20
mcg/1 mg; Phase 2:
30 mcg/1 mg; Phase
3: 35 mcg/1 mg

ETHINYL ESTRADIOL/ NORGESTIMATE

ETH in il es tra DYE
ole/nor JES ti mate

TRADE NAME(S):
Ortho-Cyclen

THERAPEUTIC CLASS:
Contraceptive
(monophasic)

GENERAL USES:
Contraception

DOSAGE FORMS:
Tablets: 35 mcg/0.25
mg

ETHINYL ESTRADIOL/ NORGESTIMATE

ETH in il es tra DYE
ole/nor JES ti mate

TRADE NAME(S):
Ortho-Tri-Cyclen

THERAPEUTIC CLASS:
Contraceptive (triphasic)

GENERAL USES:
Contraception

DOSAGE FORMS:
Tablets: Phase 1: 35
mcg/0.18 mg; Phase
2: 35 mcg/0.215 mg;
Phase 3: 35 mcg/0.25
mg

ETHINYL ESTRADIOL/ NORGESTREL

ETH in il es tra DYE

ole/nor JES trel
TRADE NAME(S):
Ovral
THERAPEUTIC CLASS:
Contraceptive
(monophasic)
GENERAL USES:
Contraception
DOSAGE FORMS:
Tablets: 50 mcg/0.5
mg

ETHINYL ESTRADIOL/ NORGESTREL
ETH in il es tra DYE
ole/nor JES trel
TRADE NAME(S):
Lo/Ovral
THERAPEUTIC CLASS:
Contraceptive
(monophasic)
GENERAL USES:
Contraception
DOSAGE FORMS:
Tablets: 30 mcg/0.3 mg

ETHIONAMIDE
e thye on AM ide
TRADE NAME(S):
Trecator-SC
THERAPEUTIC CLASS:
Antituberculosis agent
GENERAL USES:
Tuberculosis
DOSAGE FORMS:

Tablets: 250 mg

ETHOSUXIMIDE
eth oh SUKS i mide
TRADE NAME(S):
Zarontin
THERAPEUTIC CLASS:
Anticonvulsant
GENERAL USES:
Seizures
DOSAGE FORMS:
Capsules: 250 mg;
Syrup: 250 mg/5 mL

ETIDRONATE
e ti DROE nate
TRADE NAME(S):
Didronel
THERAPEUTIC CLASS:
Bisphosphonate
GENERAL USES:
Paget's disease,
hypercalcemia (cancer
related)
DOSAGE FORMS:
Tablets: 200 mg, 400 mg

ETODOLAC
ee toe DOE lak
TRADE NAME(S):
Lodine, Lodine XL
THERAPEUTIC CLASS:
Anti-inflammatory/
analgesic

GENERAL USES:
Osteoarthritis, rheumatoid arthritis, ankylosing spondylitis, pain

DOSAGE FORMS:
Tablets: 400 mg, 500 mg; Extended release tablets: 400 mg, 500 mg, 600 mg; Capsules: 200 mg, 300 mg

ETRETINATE
ee TRET ih nate

TRADE NAME(S):
Tegison

THERAPEUTIC CLASS:
Retinoid

GENERAL USES:
Psoriasis

DOSAGE FORMS:
Capsules: 10 mg, 25 mg

EXEMESTANE
ex e MES tane

TRADE NAME(S):
Aromasin

THERAPEUTIC CLASS:
Antineoplastic

GENERAL USES:
Breast cancer

DOSAGE FORMS:
Tablets: 25 mg

EZETIMIBE
ez ET i mibe

TRADE NAME(S):
Zetia

THERAPEUTIC CLASS:
Antilipemic

GENERAL USES:
Hyperlipidemia

DOSAGE FORMS:
Tablets: 10 mg

FAMCICLOVIR
fam SYE kloe veer

TRADE NAME(S):
Famvir

THERAPEUTIC CLASS:
Antiviral

GENERAL USES:
Herpes, shingles

DOSAGE FORMS:
Tablets: 125 mg, 250 mg, 500 mg

FAMOTIDINE
fa MOE ti deen

TRADE NAME(S):
Pepcid, Pepcid AC, Pepcid RPD

THERAPEUTIC CLASS:
Gastric acid secretion inhibitor

GENERAL USES:
GERD, GI ulcers

DOSAGE FORMS:
Tablets: 10 mg, 20

mg, 40 mg; Chewable
tablets: 10 mg;
Suspension: 40 mg/5
mL; Injection: 20 mg,
40 mg

FELODIPINE
fe LOE di peen
TRADE NAME(S):
Plendil
THERAPEUTIC CLASS:
Antihypertensive
GENERAL USES:
Hypertension
DOSAGE FORMS:
Extended release
tablets: 2.5 mg, 5 mg,
10 mg

FENOFIBRATE
fen oh FYE brate
TRADE NAME(S):
TriCor
THERAPEUTIC CLASS:
Antilipemic
GENERAL USES:
Hyperlipidemia
DOSAGE FORMS:
Capsules: 67 mg, 200
mg; Tablets: 54 mg,
160 mg

FENOPROFEN
fen oh PROE fen

TRADE NAME(S):
Nalfon
THERAPEUTIC CLASS:
Anti-inflammatory/
analgesic
GENERAL USES:
Osteoarthritis, rheuma-
toid arthritis, pain
DOSAGE FORMS:
Capsules: 200 mg,
300 mg; Tablets: 600
mg

FENTANYL
(INJECTION)
FEN ta nil
TRADE NAME(S):
Sublimaze
THERAPEUTIC CLASS:
Analgesic (narcotic)
GENERAL USES:
Premedicant for anes-
thesia
DOSAGE FORMS:
Injection: 0.1 mg, 0.25
mg, 0.5 mg, 1 mg, 1.5
mg, 2.5 mg

FENTANYL (ORAL)
FEN ta nil
TRADE NAME(S):
Actiq, Oralet
THERAPEUTIC CLASS:
Analgesic (narcotic)
GENERAL USES:

Pain, pre-op medication

DOSAGE FORMS:
Lozenge: 100 mcg,
200 mcg, 300 mcg,
400 mcg; Lozenge/
stick: 100 mcg, 200
mcg, 300 mcg, 400
mcg, 600 mcg, 800
mcg, 1200 mcg, 1600
mcg

FENTANYL (TRANSDERMAL)
FEN ta nil

TRADE NAME(S):
Duragesic

THERAPEUTIC CLASS:
Analgesic (narcotic)

GENERAL USES:
Pain

DOSAGE FORMS:
Transdermal patch
(mcg/hr): 25, 50, 75,
100

FEXOFENADINE
feks oh FEN a deen

TRADE NAME(S):
Allegra

THERAPEUTIC CLASS:
Antihistamine

GENERAL USES:
Allergic rhinitis

DOSAGE FORMS:
Capsules: 60 mg;
Tablets: 30 mg, 60
mg, 180 mg

FEXOFENADINE/ PSEUDOEPHEDRINE
feks oh FEN a deen/soo
doe e FED rin

TRADE NAME(S):
Allegra-D

THERAPEUTIC CLASS:
Antihistamine/
decongestant

GENERAL USES:
Allergic rhinitis

DOSAGE FORMS:
Tablets: 60 mg/120 mg

FINASTERIDE
fi NAS teer ide

TRADE NAME(S):
Propecia, Proscar

THERAPEUTIC CLASS:
Antiandrogen

GENERAL USES:
Male pattern baldness,
benign prostatic
hypertrophy

DOSAGE FORMS:
Tablets: 1 mg, 5 mg

FLECAINIDE
fle KAY nide

TRADE NAME(S):
Tambocor

THERAPEUTIC CLASS:
  Antiarrhythmic
GENERAL USES:
  Atrial fibrillation, tachy-
  cardia, arrhythmias
DOSAGE FORMS:
  Tablets: 50 mg, 100
  mg, 150 mg

FLUCONAZOLE
floo KOE na zole
TRADE NAME(S):
  Diflucan, Diflucan IV
THERAPEUTIC CLASS:
  Antifungal
GENERAL USES:
  Fungal infections
DOSAGE FORMS:
  Tablets: 50 mg, 100
  mg, 150 mg, 200 mg;
  Suspension: 10 mg/mL,
  40 mg/mL; Injection:
  200 mg, 400 mg

FLUCYTOSINE
floo SYE toe seen
TRADE NAME(S):
  Ancobon
THERAPEUTIC CLASS:
  Antifungal
GENERAL USES:
  Fungal infections
DOSAGE FORMS:
  Capsules: 250 mg,
  500 mg

FLUNISOLIDE
(INHALED)
floo NISS oh lide
TRADE NAME(S):
  AeroBid
THERAPEUTIC CLASS:
  Corticosteroid (inhaler)
GENERAL USES:
  Asthma (chronic)
DOSAGE FORMS:
  Inhaler: 250 mcg/
  inhalation

FLUNISOLIDE
(NASAL)
floo NISS oh lide
TRADE NAME(S):
  Nasalide, Nasarel
THERAPEUTIC CLASS:
  Corticosteroid (nasal)
GENERAL USES:
  Allergies
DOSAGE FORMS:
  Nasal spray: 0.025%

FLUOCINOLONE
floo oh SIN oh lone
TRADE NAME(S):
  Synalar, Fluonid,
  Flurosyn
THERAPEUTIC CLASS:
  Corticosteroid (topical)
GENERAL USES:
  Various skin conditions
DOSAGE FORMS:

Ointment: 0.025%;
Cream: 0.01%,
0.025%, 0.2%;
Solution: 0.01%

FLUOCINONIDE
floo oh SIN oh nide
TRADE NAME(S):
Lidex, Fluonex
THERAPEUTIC CLASS:
Corticosteroid (topical)
GENERAL USES:
Various skin conditions
DOSAGE FORMS:
Cream, Ointment,
Solution, Gel: 0.05%

FLUOROMETHOLONE
flure oh METH oh lone
TRADE NAME(S):
Fluor-Op, FML, Flarex
THERAPEUTIC CLASS:
Ocular agent (steroid)
GENERAL USES:
Ocular inflammation
DOSAGE FORMS:
Ophthalmic
suspension: 0.1%,
0.25%; Ophthalmic
ointment: 0.1%

FLUOROURACIL
(INJECTION)
flure oh YOOR a sil
TRADE NAME(S):
Adrucil, 5-FU
THERAPEUTIC CLASS:
Antineoplastic
GENERAL USES:
Cancers of the colon,
rectum, breast, stom-
ach, and pancreas
DOSAGE FORMS:
Injection: 500 mg, 1 g,
2.5 g, 5 g

FLUOROURACIL
(TOPICAL)
flure oh YOOR a sil
TRADE NAME(S):
Efudex, Fluoroplex
THERAPEUTIC CLASS:
Antineoplastic
GENERAL USES:
Skin disorders
DOSAGE FORMS:
Cream: 1%, 5%;
Solution: 1%, 2%, 5%

FLUOXETINE
floo OKS e teen
TRADE NAME(S):
Prozac, Prozac
Weekly, Sarafem
THERAPEUTIC CLASS:
Antidepressant
GENERAL USES:
Depression, bulimia,
obsessive-compulsive

disorder, premenstrual
dysphoric disorder

DOSAGE FORMS:
Capsules: 10 mg, 20
mg, 40 mg; Solution:
20 mg/5 mL; Delayed
release capsules: 90
mg

FLUPHENAZINE
floo FEN a zeen

TRADE NAME(S):
Prolixin, Permitil

THERAPEUTIC CLASS:
Antipsychotic

GENERAL USES:
Psychotic disorders

DOSAGE FORMS:
Tablets: 1 mg, 2.5 mg,
5 mg, 10 mg; Elixir:
2.5 mg/5 mL;
Concentrated solution:
5 mg/mL

FLURAZEPAM
flure AZ e pam

TRADE NAME(S):
Dalmane

THERAPEUTIC CLASS:
Sedative/hypnotic

GENERAL USES:
Insomnia

DOSAGE FORMS:
Capsules: 15 mg, 30
mg

FLURBIPROFEN
(OCULAR)
flur BI proe fen

TRADE NAME(S):
Ocufen

THERAPEUTIC CLASS:
Ocular agent

GENERAL USES:
Maintain pupil dilation
during surgery

DOSAGE FORMS:
Ophthalmic solution:
0.03%

FLURBIPROFEN
(ORAL)
flur BI proe fen

TRADE NAME(S):
Ansaid

THERAPEUTIC CLASS:
Anti-inflammatory/
analgesic

GENERAL USES:
Osteoarthritis, rheuma-
toid arthritis

DOSAGE FORMS:
Tablets: 50 mg, 100 mg

FLUTAMIDE
FLOO ta mide

TRADE NAME(S):
Eulexin

THERAPEUTIC CLASS:
Antiandrogen/antineo-
plastic

GENERAL USES:
Prostate cancer
DOSAGE FORMS:
Capsules: 125 mg

FLUTICASONE (INHALED)

floo TIK a sone
TRADE NAME(S):
Flovent
THERAPEUTIC CLASS:
Corticosteroid (inhaler)
GENERAL USES:
Asthma (chronic)
DOSAGE FORMS:
Inhaler:
44 mcg/inhalation,
110 mcg/inhalation,
220 mcg/inhalation

FLUTICASONE (NASAL)

floo TIK a sone
TRADE NAME(S):
Flonase
THERAPEUTIC CLASS:
Corticosteroid (nasal)
GENERAL USES:
Allergies
DOSAGE FORMS:
Nasal spray: 0.05%

FLUTICASONE PROPIONATE (TOPICAL)

floo TIK a sone
TRADE NAME(S):
Cutivate
THERAPEUTIC CLASS:
Corticosteroid (topical)
GENERAL USES:
Various skin conditions
DOSAGE FORMS:
Cream: 0.05%;
Ointment: 0.005%

FLUTICASONE/ SALMETEROL

floo TIK a sone/sal ME
te role
TRADE NAME(S):
Advair Diskus
THERAPEUTIC CLASS:
Corticosteroid/bron-
chodilator
GENERAL USES:
Asthma (chronic)
DOSAGE FORMS:
Inhalation: 0.1
mg/0.05 mg/inhala-
tion, 0.25 mg/0.05
mg/inhalation, 0.5
mg/0.05 mg/inhalation

FLUVASTATIN

FLOO va sta tin

TRADE NAME(S):
Lescol

THERAPEUTIC CLASS:
Antilipemic

GENERAL USES:
Hyperlipidemia

DOSAGE FORMS:
Capsules: 20 mg, 40 mg;
Extended release tablets:
80 mg

FLUVOXAMINE
floo VOKS a meen

TRADE NAME(S):
Luvox

THERAPEUTIC CLASS:
Antidepressant

GENERAL USES:
Obsessive-compulsive
disorder

DOSAGE FORMS:
Tablets: 25 mg, 50
mg, 100 mg

FONDAPARINUX SODIUM
fon da PARE i nuks

TRADE NAME(S):
Arixtra

THERAPEUTIC CLASS:
Anticoagulant (LMWH)

GENERAL USES:
Prevention of blood
clots

DOSAGE FORMS:
Injection: 2.5 mg

FORMOTEROL
for MOH te rol

TRADE NAME(S):
Foradil

THERAPEUTIC CLASS:
Bronchodilator

GENERAL USES:
Asthma (chronic)

DOSAGE FORMS:
Inhalation: 12
mcg/inhalation

FOSCARNET
fos KAR net

TRADE NAME(S):
Foscavir

THERAPEUTIC CLASS:
Antiviral

GENERAL USES:
CMV retinitis, herpes
simplex virus infections

DOSAGE FORMS:
Injection: 6 g, 12 g

FOSINOPRIL
foe SIN oh pril

TRADE NAME(S):
Monopril

THERAPEUTIC CLASS:
Antihypertensive, cardiac agent

GENERAL USES:
Hypertension, heart
failure
DOSAGE FORMS:
Tablets: 10 mg,
20 mg, 40 mg

FOSPHENYTOIN
FOS fen i toyn
TRADE NAME(S):
Cerebyx
THERAPEUTIC CLASS:
Anticonvulsants
GENERAL USES:
Seizures
DOSAGE FORMS:
Injection: 150 mg,
750 mg

FROVATRIPTAN
froe va TRIP tan
TRADE NAME(S):
Frova
THERAPEUTIC CLASS:
Antimigraine agent
GENERAL USES:
Acute treatment of
migraine
DOSAGE FORMS:
Tablets: 2.5 mg

FUROSEMIDE
fyoor OH se mide
TRADE NAME(S):
Lasix
THERAPEUTIC CLASS:
Diuretic
GENERAL USES:
CHF & pulmonary
related edema, hyper-
tension
DOSAGE FORMS:
Tablets: 20 mg, 40 mg,
80 mg; Solution: 10
mg/mL, 40 mg/5 mL;
Injection: 20 mg, 40
mg, 100 mg

GABAPENTIN
GA ba pen tin
TRADE NAME(S):
Neurontin
THERAPEUTIC CLASS:
Anticonvulsant
GENERAL USES:
Seizures
DOSAGE FORMS:
Capsules: 100 mg,
300 mg, 400 mg;
Tablets: 600 mg, 800
mg; Solution: 250
mg/5 mL

GALANTAMINE
ga LAN ta meen
TRADE NAME(S):
Reminyl
THERAPEUTIC CLASS:
Alzheimer's agent

GENERAL USES:
Mild to moderate
dementia of
Alzheimer's
DOSAGE FORMS:
Tablets: 4 mg, 8 mg,
12 mg; Solution: 4
mg/mL

GANCICLOVIR
gan SYE kloe veer
TRADE NAME(S):
Cytovene
THERAPEUTIC CLASS:
Antiviral
GENERAL USES:
CMV retinitis & infec-
tion
DOSAGE FORMS:
Capsules: 250 mg,
500 mg; Injection: 500
mg

GATIFLOXACIN
gat i FLOKS a sin
TRADE NAME(S):
Tequin
THERAPEUTIC CLASS:
Anti-infective
GENERAL USES:
Bacterial infections
DOSAGE FORMS:
Tablets: 200 mg, 400
mg; Injection: 200 mg,
400 mg

GEMFIBROZIL
jem FI broe zil
TRADE NAME(S):
Lopid
THERAPEUTIC CLASS:
Antilipemic
GENERAL USES:
Hyperlipidemia
DOSAGE FORMS:
Tablets: 600 mg

GEMTUZUMAB OZOGAMICIN
gem TOO zoo mab oh
zog a MY sin
TRADE NAME(S):
Mylotarg
THERAPEUTIC CLASS:
Antineoplastic
GENERAL USES:
Acute myeloid
leukemia
DOSAGE FORMS:
Injection: 5 mg

GENTAMICIN
jen ta MYE sin
TRADE NAME(S):
Garamycin, Genoptic,
Gentak
THERAPEUTIC CLASS:
Ocular agent (anti-
infective)
GENERAL USES:
Ocular infections

DOSAGE FORMS:
Ophthalmic ointment:
3 mg/g; Ophthalmic
solution: 3 mg/mL

GENTAMICIN (INJECTION)
jen ta MYE sin
TRADE NAME(S):
Garamycin
THERAPEUTIC CLASS:
Anti-infective
GENERAL USES:
Bacterial infections
DOSAGE FORMS:
Injection: 20 mg, 60
mg, 80 mg, 800 mg

GLIMEPIRIDE
GLYE me pye ride
TRADE NAME(S):
Amaryl
THERAPEUTIC CLASS:
Antidiabetic
GENERAL USES:
Diabetes (type 2)
DOSAGE FORMS:
Tablets: 1 mg, 2 mg, 4
mg

GLIPIZIDE
GLIP i zide
TRADE NAME(S):
Glucotrol, Glucotrol XL

THERAPEUTIC CLASS:
Antidiabetic
GENERAL USES:
Diabetes (type 2)
DOSAGE FORMS:
Tablets & Extended
release tablets: 5 mg,
10 mg

GLYBURIDE
GLYE byoor ide
TRADE NAME(S):
Diabeta, Micronase,
Glynase
THERAPEUTIC CLASS:
Antidiabetic
GENERAL USES:
Diabetes (type 2)
DOSAGE FORMS:
Tablets: 1.25 mg, 2.5
mg, 5 mg; Micronized
tablets: 1.5 mg, 3 mg,
4.5 mg, 6 mg

GLYBURIDE/ METFORMIN
GLYE byoor ide/met
FOR min
TRADE NAME(S):
Glucovance
THERAPEUTIC CLASS:
Antidiabetic
GENERAL USES:
Diabetes (type 2)

DOSAGE FORMS:
Tablets: 1.25 mg/250 mg, 2.5 mg/500 mg, 5 mg/500 mg

GRANISETRON
gra NI se tron
TRADE NAME(S):
Kytril
THERAPEUTIC CLASS:
Antiemetic
GENERAL USES:
Chemotherapy nausea/vomiting
DOSAGE FORMS:
Tablets: 1 mg; Injection: 1 mg, 4 mg

GRISEOFULVIN MICROSIZE
gri see oh FUL vin
TRADE NAME(S):
Fulvicin, Grifulvin
THERAPEUTIC CLASS:
Antifungal
GENERAL USES:
Fungal infections
DOSAGE FORMS:
Tablets: 250 mg, 500 mg; Capsules: 125 mg, 250 mg; Suspension: 125 mg/5 mL

GRISEOFULVIN ULTRAMICROSIZE
gri see oh FUL vin
TRADE NAME(S):
Fulvicin P/G, Grisactin, Gris-PEG
THERAPEUTIC CLASS:
Antifungal
GENERAL USES:
Fungal infections
DOSAGE FORMS:
Tablets: 125 mg, 165 mg, 250 mg, 330 mg

GUANABENZ
GWAHN a benz
TRADE NAME(S):
Wytensin
THERAPEUTIC CLASS:
Antihypertensive
GENERAL USES:
Hypertension
DOSAGE FORMS:
Tablets: 4 mg, 8 mg

GUANADREL
GWAHN a drel
TRADE NAME(S):
Hylorel
THERAPEUTIC CLASS:
Antihypertensive
GENERAL USES:
Hypertension
DOSAGE FORMS:
Tablets: 10 mg, 25 mg

GUANETHIDINE
gwahn ETH i deen
TRADE NAME(S):
  Ismelin
THERAPEUTIC CLASS:
  Antihypertensive
GENERAL USES:
  Hypertension
DOSAGE FORMS:
  Tablets: 10 mg, 25 mg

GUANFACINE
GWAHN fa seen
TRADE NAME(S):
  Tenex
THERAPEUTIC CLASS:
  Antihypertensive
GENERAL USES:
  Hypertension
DOSAGE FORMS:
  Tablets: 1 mg, 2 mg

HALAZEPAM
hal AZ e pam
TRADE NAME(S):
  Paxipam
THERAPEUTIC CLASS:
  Antianxiety agent
GENERAL USES:
  Anxiety
DOSAGE FORMS:
  Tablets: 20 mg, 40 mg

HALCINONIDE
hal SIN oh nide
TRADE NAME(S):
  Halog, Halog-E
THERAPEUTIC CLASS:
  Corticosteroid
  (topical)
GENERAL USES:
  Various skin conditions
DOSAGE FORMS:
  Ointment, Solution &
  Cream: 0.1%; Cream:
  0.025%

HALOFANTRINE
ha loe FAN trin
TRADE NAME(S):
  Halfan
THERAPEUTIC CLASS:
  Antimalarial
GENERAL USES:
  Malaria treatment
DOSAGE FORMS:
  Tablets: 250 mg

HALOPERIDOL
ha loe PER i dole
TRADE NAME(S):
  Haldol
THERAPEUTIC CLASS:
  Antipsychotic
GENERAL USES:
  Psychotic/behavioral
  disorders, Tourette's

DOSAGE FORMS:
Tablets: 0.5 mg, 1 mg,
2 mg, 5 mg, 10 mg,
20 mg; Concentrated
solution: 2 mg/mL;
Injection: 5 mg, 50
mg, 100 mg, 250 mg,
500 mg

HALOPROGIN
ha loe PROE jin
TRADE NAME(S):
Halotex
THERAPEUTIC CLASS:
Antifungal (topical)
GENERAL USES:
Athlete's foot, jock
itch, ringworm, tinea
versicolor
DOSAGE FORMS:
Cream & Solution: 1%

HEPARIN
HEP a rin
TRADE NAME(S):
Heparin
THERAPEUTIC CLASS:
Anticoagulant
GENERAL USES:
Prevention of blood
clots
DOSAGE FORMS:
Various concentrations

HETASTARCH
HET a starch
TRADE NAME(S):
Hespan
THERAPEUTIC CLASS:
Plasma expander
GENERAL USES:
Shock
DOSAGE FORMS:
Injection: 30 g

HYDRALAZINE
hye DRAL a zeen
TRADE NAME(S):
Apresoline
THERAPEUTIC CLASS:
Antihypertensive
GENERAL USES:
Hypertension
DOSAGE FORMS:
Tablets: 10 mg, 25
mg, 50 mg, 100 mg;
Injection: 20 mg

HYDRALAZINE/HCTZ
hye DRAL a zeen/hye
droe klor oh THYE a zide
TRADE NAME(S):
Apresazide
THERAPEUTIC CLASS:
Antihypertensive/
diuretic
GENERAL USES:
Hypertension

DOSAGE FORMS:
  Tablets: 25 mg/25 mg, 50 mg/50 mg, 100 mg/50 mg

HYDROCHLORO-THIAZIDE
hye droe klor oh THYE a zide
TRADE NAME(S):
  Esidrix, HydroDIURIL, Oretic
THERAPEUTIC CLASS:
  Diuretic
GENERAL USES:
  CHF related edema, hypertension
DOSAGE FORMS:
  Tablets: 25 mg, 50 mg, 100 mg; Capsules: 12.5 mg; Solution: 50 mg/5 mL

HYDROCORTISONE (ORAL)
hye droe KOR ti sone
TRADE NAME(S):
  Cortef
THERAPEUTIC CLASS:
  Glucocorticoid
GENERAL USES:
  Endocrine, skin, blood disorders

DOSAGE FORMS:
  Tablets: 5 mg, 10 mg, 20 mg

HYDROCORTISONE (TOPICAL)
hye droe KOR ti sone
TRADE NAME(S):
  Hycort, Cort-Dome, Dermacort, many others
THERAPEUTIC CLASS:
  Corticosteroid (topical)
GENERAL USES:
  Various skin conditions
DOSAGE FORMS:
  Ointment, Lotion & Cream: 0.5%, 1%, 2.5%; Lotion: 2%; Gel, Solution & Spray: 1%

HYDROCORTISONE ACETATE
hye droe KOR ti sone
TRADE NAME(S):
  Hydrocortone acetate
THERAPEUTIC CLASS:
  Glucocorticoid
GENERAL USES:
  Endocrine, skin, blood disorders
DOSAGE FORMS:
  Injection: 125 mg, 250 mg, 500 mg

HYDROCORTISONE SODIUM SUCCINATE

hye droe KOR ti sone

TRADE NAME(S):
Solu-Cortef, A-Hydrocort

THERAPEUTIC CLASS:
Glucocorticoid

GENERAL USES:
Endocrine, skin, blood disorders

DOSAGE FORMS:
Injection: 100 mg, 250 mg, 500 mg, 1000 mg

HYDROXY-AMPHETAMINE

hye droks ee am FET a meen

TRADE NAME(S):
Paredrine

THERAPEUTIC CLASS:
Ocular agent

GENERAL USES:
Pupil dilation

DOSAGE FORMS:
Ophthalmic solution: 1%

HYDROXY-CHLOROQUINE

hye droks ee KLOR oh kwin

TRADE NAME(S):
Plaquenil

THERAPEUTIC CLASS:
Antirheumatic agent

GENERAL USES:
Rheumatoid arthritis, systemic lupus erythematosus

DOSAGE FORMS:
Tablets: 200 mg

HYDROXYZINE

hye DROKS i zeen

TRADE NAME(S):
Atarax, Vistaril

THERAPEUTIC CLASS:
Antihistamine

GENERAL USES:
Itching, sedation

DOSAGE FORMS:
Tablets: 10 mg, 25 mg, 50 mg, 100 mg; Capsules: 25 mg, 50 mg, 100 mg; Syrup: 10 mg/5 mL; Suspension: 25 mg/5 mL; Injection: 25 mg, 50 mg

IBUPROFEN

eye byoo PROE fen

TRADE NAME(S):
Motrin, Advil, Nuprin, many others

THERAPEUTIC CLASS:
Analgesic, antipyretic, anti-inflammatory

GENERAL USES:
  Pain, fever, arthritis
DOSAGE FORMS:
  Tablets: 100 mg, 200 mg, 300 mg, 400 mg, 600 mg, 800 mg; Chewable tablets: 50 mg, 100 mg; Capsules: 200 mg; Liquid or Suspension: 100 mg/5 mL; Suspension: 100 mg/2.5 mL; Drops: 40 mg/mL

IDOXURIDINE
eye dox YOOR i deen
TRADE NAME(S):
  Herplex
THERAPEUTIC CLASS:
  Ocular agent (antiviral)
GENERAL USES:
  Ocular herpes infections
DOSAGE FORMS:
  Ophthalmic solution: 0.1%

IMATINIB
eye MAT eh nib
TRADE NAME(S):
  Gleevec
THERAPEUTIC CLASS:
  Antineoplastic

GENERAL USES:
  Chronic myeloid leukemia
DOSAGE FORMS:
  Capsules: 100 mg

IMIPENEM/ CILASTATIN
i mi PEN em/sye la STAT in
TRADE NAME(S):
  Primaxin
THERAPEUTIC CLASS:
  Anti-infective
GENERAL USES:
  Bacterial infections
DOSAGE FORMS:
  Injection: 250 mg/250 mg, 500 mg/500 mg, 750 mg/750 mg

IMIPRAMINE HCL
im IP ra meen
TRADE NAME(S):
  Tofranil
THERAPEUTIC CLASS:
  Antidepressant
GENERAL USES:
  Depression, childhood bedwetting
DOSAGE FORMS:
  Tablets: 10 mg, 25 mg, 50 mg

IMIPRAMINE PAMOATE
im IP ra meen
TRADE NAME(S):
Tofranil-PM
THERAPEUTIC CLASS:
Antidepressant
GENERAL USES:
Depression
DOSAGE FORMS:
Capsules: 75 mg, 100 mg, 125 mg, 150 mg

IMIQUIMOD
i mi KWI mod
TRADE NAME(S):
Aldara
THERAPEUTIC CLASS:
Immunomodulator (topical)
GENERAL USES:
Genital and anal warts
DOSAGE FORMS:
Cream: 5%

INDAPAMIDE
in DAP a mide
TRADE NAME(S):
Lozol
THERAPEUTIC CLASS:
Diuretic
GENERAL USES:
CHF, hypertension
DOSAGE FORMS:
Tablets: 1.25 mg, 2.5 mg

INDINAVIR
in DIN a veer
TRADE NAME(S):
Crixivan
THERAPEUTIC CLASS:
Antiviral
GENERAL USES:
HIV infection
DOSAGE FORMS:
Capsules: 100 mg, 200 mg, 333 mg, 400 mg

INDOMETHACIN
in doe METH a sin
TRADE NAME(S):
Indocin, Indocin ER, Indocin SR
THERAPEUTIC CLASS:
Anti-inflammatory/ analgesic
GENERAL USES:
Various arthritis conditions, pain
DOSAGE FORMS:
Capsules: 25 mg, 50 mg; Sustained release capsules: 75 mg; Suspension: 25 mg/5 mL

INSULIN
IN su lin
TRADE NAME(S):
Iletin II, Novolin R, Humulin R

THERAPEUTIC CLASS:
  Antidiabetic
GENERAL USES:
  Diabetes
DOSAGE FORMS:
  Injection: 100 units/mL

INSULIN, ANALOG
IN su lin
TRADE NAME(S):
  Humalog, Humalog
  Mix 75/25, NovoLog
THERAPEUTIC CLASS:
  Antidiabetic
GENERAL USES:
  Diabetes
DOSAGE FORMS:
  Injection: 100 units/mL

INSULIN, ASPART
IN su lin
TRADE NAME(S):
  NovoLog
THERAPEUTIC CLASS:
  Antidiabetic
GENERAL USES:
  Diabetes
DOSAGE FORMS:
  Injection: 100 units/mL

INSULIN, GLARGINE
IN su lin
TRADE NAME(S):
  Lantus

THERAPEUTIC CLASS:
  Antidiabetic
GENERAL USES:
  Diabetes
DOSAGE FORMS:
  Injection: 100 units/mL

INSULIN, ISOPHANE SUSPENSION
IN su lin
TRADE NAME(S):
  NPH Iletin, Novolin N,
  Humulin N
THERAPEUTIC CLASS:
  Antidiabetic
GENERAL USES:
  Diabetes
DOSAGE FORMS:
  Injection: 100
  units/mL

INSULIN, ISOPHANE AND INSULIN SUSPENSION
IN su lin
TRADE NAME(S):
  Humulin 50/50,
  Novolin 70/30,
  Humulin 70/30
THERAPEUTIC CLASS:
  Antidiabetic
GENERAL USES:
  Diabetes
DOSAGE FORMS:
  Injection: 100 units/mL

INSULIN, ZINC SUSPENSION

IN su lin

TRADE NAME(S):
Lente Iletin II, Humulin L, Novolin L

THERAPEUTIC CLASS:
Antidiabetic

GENERAL USES:
Diabetes

DOSAGE FORMS:
Injection: 100 units/mL

INSULIN, ZINC SUSPENSION, EXTENDED

IN su lin

TRADE NAME(S):
Humulin U

THERAPEUTIC CLASS:
Antidiabetic

GENERAL USES:
Diabetes

DOSAGE FORMS:
Injection: 100 units/mL

INTERFERON ALFA-2a

in ter FEER on

TRADE NAME(S):
Roferon-A

THERAPEUTIC CLASS:
Immune modulator

GENERAL USES:
Leukemia, AIDS sarcoma

DOSAGE FORMS:
Injection: 3 million IU, 6 million IU, 9 million IU, 18 million IU, 36 million IU

INTERFERON ALFA-2b

in ter FEER on

TRADE NAME(S):
Intron-A

THERAPEUTIC CLASS:
Immune modulator

GENERAL USES:
Leukemia, AIDS sarcoma, Hepatitis B, C (chronic)

DOSAGE FORMS:
Injection: 3 million IU, 5 million IU, 10 million IU, 18 million IU, 25 million IU, 50 million IU

INTERFERON BETA-1a

in ter FEER on

TRADE NAME(S):
Avonex

THERAPEUTIC CLASS:
Immune modulator

GENERAL USES:
Multiple sclerosis

DOSAGE FORMS:
Injection: 6.6 million IU (33 mcg)

INTERFERON BETA-1b
in ter FEER on
TRADE NAME(S):
Betaseron
THERAPEUTIC CLASS:
Immune modulator
GENERAL USES:
Multiple sclerosis
DOSAGE FORMS:
Injection: 9.6 million IU (0.3 mg)

IODOQUINOL
eye oh doe KWIN ole
TRADE NAME(S):
Yodoxin
THERAPEUTIC CLASS:
Antituberculosis agent
GENERAL USES:
Tuberculosis
DOSAGE FORMS:
Tablets: 210 mg, 650 mg; Powder: 25 g

IPRATROPIUM
i pra TROE pee´um
TRADE NAME(S):
Atrovent
THERAPEUTIC CLASS:
Bronchodilator

GENERAL USES:
Bronchospasm, asthma
DOSAGE FORMS:
Inhalation solution: 0.02%; Inhaler: 18 mcg/inhalation; Nasal spray: 0.03%, 0.06%

IPRATROPIUM/ ALBUTEROL
i pra TROE pee um/al BYOO ter ole
TRADE NAME(S):
Combivent
THERAPEUTIC CLASS:
Bronchodilator
GENERAL USES:
Bronchospasm
DOSAGE FORMS:
Inhaler: 18 mcg/103 mcg/inhalation

IRBESARTAN
ir be SAR tan
TRADE NAME(S):
Avapro
THERAPEUTIC CLASS:
Antihypertensive
GENERAL USES:
Hypertension
DOSAGE FORMS:
Tablets: 75 mg, 150 mg, 300 mg

ISOCARBOXAZID

eye so car BOX ah zid

TRADE NAME(S):
Marplan

THERAPEUTIC CLASS:
Antidepressant

GENERAL USES:
Depression

DOSAGE FORMS:
Tablets: 10 mg

ISOETHARINE

eye soe ETH a reen

TRADE NAME(S):
Bronkosol

THERAPEUTIC CLASS:
Bronchodilator

GENERAL USES:
Bronchospasm, asthma

DOSAGE FORMS:
Inhalation solution: 1%

ISONIAZID

eye soe NYE a zid

TRADE NAME(S):
Laniazid, Nydrazid

THERAPEUTIC CLASS:
Antituberculosis agent

GENERAL USES:
Tuberculosis

DOSAGE FORMS:
Tablets: 50 mg, 100 mg, 300 mg; Syrup: 50 mg/5 mL; Injection: 1 g

ISOPROTERENOL

eye soe proe TER e nole

TRADE NAME(S):
Isuprel, Medihaler

THERAPEUTIC CLASS:
Bronchodilator

GENERAL USES:
Bronchospasm, asthma

DOSAGE FORMS:
Inhalation solution: 0.5%, 1%; Inhaler: 103 mcg/inhalation, 80 mcg/inhalation

ISOSORBIDE DINITRATE

eye soe SOR bide dye NYE trate

TRADE NAME(S):
Isordil, Sorbitrate

THERAPEUTIC CLASS:
Antianginal

GENERAL USES:
Angina

DOSAGE FORMS:
Tablets: 5 mg, 10 mg, 20 mg, 30 mg, 40 mg; Sustained release tablets & capsules: 40 mg; Sublingual tablets: 2.5 mg, 5 mg, 10 mg; Chewable tablets: 5 mg, 10 mg

ISOSORBIDE MONONITRATE
eye soe SOR bide mon oh NYE trate

TRADE NAME(S):
Ismo, Monoket, Imdur

THERAPEUTIC CLASS:
Antianginal

GENERAL USES:
Angina

DOSAGE FORMS:
Tablets: 10 mg, 20 mg; Extended release tablets: 30 mg, 60 mg, 120 mg

ISOTRETINOIN
eye soe TRET i noyn

TRADE NAME(S):
Accutane

THERAPEUTIC CLASS:
Retinoid

GENERAL USES:
Severe cystic acne

DOSAGE FORMS:
Capsules: 10 mg, 20 mg, 40 mg

ISRADIPINE
iz RA di peen

TRADE NAME(S):
DynaCirc CR, DynaCirc

THERAPEUTIC CLASS:
Antihypertensive

GENERAL USES:
Hypertension

DOSAGE FORMS:
Capsules: 2.5 mg, 5 mg; Controlled release tablets: 5 mg, 10 mg

ITRACONAZOLE
i tra KOE na zole

TRADE NAME(S):
Sporanox

THERAPEUTIC CLASS:
Antifungal

GENERAL USES:
Fungal infections

DOSAGE FORMS:
Capsules: 100 mg; Solution: 10 mg/mL; Injection: 10 mg

KANAMYCIN
kan a MYE sin

TRADE NAME(S):
Kantrex

THERAPEUTIC CLASS:
Anti-infective

GENERAL USES:
Bacterial infections

DOSAGE FORMS:
Injection: 150 mg, 1 g, 2 g, 3 g

KETOCONAZOLE

kee toe KOE na zole

TRADE NAME(S):
Nizoral

THERAPEUTIC CLASS:
Antifungal (oral & topical)

GENERAL USES:
Fungal infections

DOSAGE FORMS:
Tablets: 200 mg;
Shampoo & Cream:
2%

KETOPROFEN

kee toe PROE fen

TRADE NAME(S):
Orudis KT, Actron,
Orudis, Oruvail

THERAPEUTIC CLASS:
Anti-inflammatory/
analgesic

GENERAL USES:
Osteoarthritis, rheumatoid arthritis, pain

DOSAGE FORMS:
Capsules: 12.5 mg, 25
mg, 50 mg, 75 mg;
Extended release capsules: 100 mg, 150
mg, 200 mg

KETOROLAC

KEE toe role ak

TRADE NAME(S):
Toradol

THERAPEUTIC CLASS:
Anti-inflammatory/
analgesic

GENERAL USES:
Severe acute pain
(short-term therapy)

DOSAGE FORMS:
Tablets: 10 mg;
Injection: 15 mg, 30
mg, 60 mg

KETOROLAC (OCULAR)

KEE toe role ak

TRADE NAME(S):
Acular

THERAPEUTIC CLASS:
Ocular agent

GENERAL USES:
Allergic conjunctivitis

DOSAGE FORMS:
Ophthalmic solution:
0.5%

KETOTIFEN

kee toe TYE fen

TRADE NAME(S):
Zaditor

THERAPEUTIC CLASS:
Ocular agent

GENERAL USES:

Allergic conjunctivitis
DOSAGE FORMS:
Ophthalmic solution:
0.025%

LABETALOL
la BET a lole
TRADE NAME(S):
Normodyne, Trandate
THERAPEUTIC CLASS:
Antihypertensive
GENERAL USES:
Hypertension
DOSAGE FORMS:
Tablets: 100 mg, 200
mg, 300 mg

LAMIVUDINE (3TC)
la MI vyoo deen
TRADE NAME(S):
Epivir, Epivir-HBV
THERAPEUTIC CLASS:
Antiviral
GENERAL USES:
HIV infection
DOSAGE FORMS:
Tablets: 100 mg, 150
mg; Solution: 5
mg/mL, 10 mg/mL

LAMIVUDINE/
ZIDOVUDINE
la MI vyoo deen/zye
DOE vyoo deen

TRADE NAME(S):
Combivir
THERAPEUTIC CLASS:
Antiviral
GENERAL USES:
HIV infection
DOSAGE FORMS:
Tablets: 150 mg/300
mg

LAMOTRIGINE
la MOE tri jeen
TRADE NAME(S):
Lamictal
THERAPEUTIC CLASS:
Anticonvulsant
GENERAL USES:
Seizures
DOSAGE FORMS:
Tablets: 25 mg, 100
mg, 150 mg, 200 mg;
Chewable tablets: 5
mg, 25 mg

LANSOPRAZOLE
lan SOE pra zole
TRADE NAME(S):
Prevacid
THERAPEUTIC CLASS:
Gastric acid secretion
inhibitor
GENERAL USES:
Duodenal ulcer, GERD

DOSAGE FORMS:
Delayed release capsules & suspension:
15 mg, 30 mg

LATANOPROST
la TA noe prost
TRADE NAME(S):
Xalatan
THERAPEUTIC CLASS:
Ocular agent
GENERAL USES:
Glaucoma/ocular hypertension
DOSAGE FORMS:
Ophthalmic solution:
0.005%

LEFLUNOMIDE
le FLOO noh mide
TRADE NAME(S):
Arava
THERAPEUTIC CLASS:
Antirheumatic
GENERAL USES:
Rhematoid arthritis
DOSAGE FORMS:
Tablets: 10 mg, 20 mg, 100 mg

LEPIRUDIN
leh puh ROO din
TRADE NAME(S):
Refludan

THERAPEUTIC CLASS:
Anticoagulant
GENERAL USES:
Heparin induced thrombocytopenia
DOSAGE FORMS:
Injection: 50 mg

LETROZOLE
LET roe zole
TRADE NAME(S):
Femara
THERAPEUTIC CLASS:
Antineoplastic
GENERAL USES:
Breast cancer
DOSAGE FORMS:
Tablets: 2.5 mg

LEVETIRACETAM
lee va tye RA se tam
TRADE NAME(S):
Keppra
THERAPEUTIC CLASS:
Anticonvulsant
GENERAL USES:
Partial seizures
DOSAGE FORMS:
Tablets: 250 mg, 500 mg, 750 mg

LEVOBETAXOLOL

lee voe be TAX oh lol

TRADE NAME(S):
Betaxon

THERAPEUTIC CLASS:
Ocular agent

GENERAL USES:
Open angle glaucoma, ocular hypertension

DOSAGE FORMS:
Ophthalmic suspension: 0.5%

LEVOBUNOLOL

lee voe BYOO noe lole

TRADE NAME(S):
AKBeta, Betagan

THERAPEUTIC CLASS:
Ocular agent

GENERAL USES:
Glaucoma/ocular hypertension

DOSAGE FORMS:
Ophthalmic solution: 0.25%, 0.5%

LEVOCABASTINE

LEE voe kab as teen

TRADE NAME(S):
Livostin

THERAPEUTIC CLASS:
Ocular agent

GENERAL USES:
Allergic conjunctivitis

DOSAGE FORMS:
Ophthalmic suspension: 0.05%

LEVODOPA/ CARBIDOPA

lee voe DOE pa/kar bi DOE pa

TRADE NAME(S):
Sinemet, Sinemet CR

THERAPEUTIC CLASS:
Antiparkinson agent

GENERAL USES:
Parkinson's disease

DOSAGE FORMS:
Tablets: 100 mg/10 mg, 100 mg/25 mg, 250 mg/25 mg; Sustained release tablets: 100 mg/25 mg, 200 mg/50 mg

LEVOFLOXACIN

lee voe FLOKS a sin

TRADE NAME(S):
Levaquin

THERAPEUTIC CLASS:
Anti-infective

GENERAL USES:
Bacterial infections

DOSAGE FORMS:
Tablets: 250 mg, 500 mg; Injection: 250 mg, 500 mg, 750 mg

LEVONORGESTREL
LEE voe nor jes trel
TRADE NAME(S):
 Plan B
THERAPEUTIC CLASS:
 Contraceptive (emergency)
GENERAL USES:
 Emergency contraception
DOSAGE FORMS:
 Tablets: 0.75 mg

LEVOTHYROXINE
lee voe thye ROKS een
TRADE NAME(S):
 Synthroid, Levothroid, Levo-T, Levoxyl
THERAPEUTIC CLASS:
 Hormone (thyroid)
GENERAL USES:
 Hypothyroidism
DOSAGE FORMS:
 Tablets: 25 mcg, 50 mcg, 75 mcg, 88 mcg, 100 mcg, 112 mcg, 125 mcg, 137 mcg, 150 mcg, 175 mcg, 200 mcg, 300 mcg; Injection: 200 mcg, 500 mcg

LIDOCAINE
LYE doe kane
TRADE NAME(S):
 Xylocaine
THERAPEUTIC CLASS:
 Antiarrhythmic
GENERAL USES:
 Arrhythmias
DOSAGE FORMS:
 Injection: 50 mg, 200 mg, 300 mg, 400 mg, 500 mg, 1 g, 2 g, 4 g

LINDANE
LIN dane
TRADE NAME(S):
 Kwell, G-well
THERAPEUTIC CLASS:
 Scabicide/pediculicide (topical)
GENERAL USES:
 Scabies, head lice
DOSAGE FORMS:
 Lotion & Shampoo: 1%

LINEZOLID
li NE zoh lid
TRADE NAME(S):
 Zyvox
THERAPEUTIC CLASS:
 Anti-infective
GENERAL USES:
 Vancomycin resistant bacterial infections
DOSAGE FORMS:

Tablets: 400 mg, 600 mg; Suspension: 100 mg/5 mL; Injection: 200 mg, 600 mg

LIOTHYRONINE
lye oh THYE roe neen

TRADE NAME(S):
Cytomel, Triostat

THERAPEUTIC CLASS:
Hormone (thyroid)

GENERAL USES:
Hypothyroidism

DOSAGE FORMS:
Tablets: 5 mcg, 25 mcg, 50 mcg; Injection: 10 mcg

LISINOPRIL
lyse IN oh pril

TRADE NAME(S):
Zestril, Prinivil

THERAPEUTIC CLASS:
Antihypertensive, cardiac agent

GENERAL USES:
Hypertension, heart failure, myocardial infarction

DOSAGE FORMS:
Tablets: 2.5 mg, 5 mg, 10 mg, 20 mg, 40 mg

LISINOPRIL/HCTZ
lyse IN oh pril/hye droe klor oh THYE a zide

TRADE NAME(S):
Zestoretic, Prinzide

THERAPEUTIC CLASS:
Antihypertensive/diuretic

GENERAL USES:
Hypertension

DOSAGE FORMS:
Tablets: 10 mg/12.5 mg, 20 mg/12.5 mg, 20 mg/25 mg

LITHIUM
LITH ee um

TRADE NAME(S):
Eskalith, Eskalith CR, Lithotabs, Lithobid

THERAPEUTIC CLASS:
Antipsychotic

GENERAL USES:
Psychotic disorders

DOSAGE FORMS:
Capsules: 150 mg, 300 mg, 600 mg; Tablets: 300 mg; Sustained release tablets: 300 mg; Controlled release tablets: 450 mg; Syrup: 8 mEq or 300 mg/5 mL

LODOXAMIDE

loe DOKS a mide

TRADE NAME(S):
Alomide

THERAPEUTIC CLASS:
Ocular agent

GENERAL USES:
Allergic conjunctivitis

DOSAGE FORMS:
Ophthalmic solution:
0.1%

LOMEFLOXACIN

loe me FLOKS a sin

TRADE NAME(S):
Maxaquin

THERAPEUTIC CLASS:
Anti-infective

GENERAL USES:
Bacterial infections

DOSAGE FORMS:
Tablets: 400 mg

LOPINAVIR/ RITONAVIR

loe PIN a veer/rit ON uh
veer

TRADE NAME(S):
Kaletra

THERAPEUTIC CLASS:
Antiviral

GENERAL USES:
HIV infection

DOSAGE FORMS:
Capsules: 133.3
mg/33.3 mg; Solution:
80 mg/20 mg per mL

LORACARBEF

lor a KAR bef

TRADE NAME(S):
Lorabid

THERAPEUTIC CLASS:
Anti-infective

GENERAL USES:
Bacterial infections

DOSAGE FORMS:
Capsules: 200 mg,
400 mg; Suspension:
100 mg/5 mL, 200
mg/5 mL

LORATADINE

lor AT a deen

TRADE NAME(S):
Claritin

THERAPEUTIC CLASS:
Antihistamine

GENERAL USES:
Allergic rhinitis/hives

DOSAGE FORMS:
Tablets: 10 mg; Syrup:
1 mg/mL (240 mL);
Rapid disintegrating
tablets: 10 mg

LORATADINE/ PSEUDOEPHEDRINE

lor AT a deen/soo doe e FED rin

TRADE NAME(S):
Claritin-D, Claritin-D 24 Hour

THERAPEUTIC CLASS:
Antihistamine/decongestant

GENERAL USES:
Allergic rhinitis

DOSAGE FORMS:
Tablets: 5 mg/120 mg (D), 10 mg/240 mg (D-24)

LORAZEPAM

lor A ze pam

TRADE NAME(S):
Ativan

THERAPEUTIC CLASS:
Antianxiety agent

GENERAL USES:
Anxiety, sedation

DOSAGE FORMS:
Tablets: 0.5 mg, 1 mg, 2 mg; Concentrated solution: 2 mg/mL; Injection: 2 mg, 4 mg, 8 mg, 20 mg, 40 mg

LOSARTAN

loe SAR tan

TRADE NAME(S):
Cozaar

THERAPEUTIC CLASS:
Antihypertensive

GENERAL USES:
Hypertension

DOSAGE FORMS:
Tablets: 25 mg, 50 mg, 100 mg

LOSARTAN/HCTZ

loe SAR tan/hye droe klor oh THYE a zide

TRADE NAME(S):
Hyzaar

THERAPEUTIC CLASS:
Antihypertensive/ diuretic

GENERAL USES:
Hypertension

DOSAGE FORMS:
Tablets: 50 mg/12.5 mg, 100 mg/25 mg

LOTEPREDNOL

loe te PRED nol

TRADE NAME(S):
Lotemax, Alrex

THERAPEUTIC CLASS:
Ocular agent

GENERAL USES:
Ocular inflammation, allergies

DOSAGE FORMS:
Ophthalmic suspension: 0.2%, 0.5%

LOVASTATIN

LOE va sta tin

TRADE NAME(S):
Mevacor

THERAPEUTIC CLASS:
Antilipemic

GENERAL USES:
Hyperlipidemia, artherosclerosis

DOSAGE FORMS:
Tablets: 10 mg, 20 mg, 40 mg; Extended release tablets: 10 mg, 20 mg, 40 mg, 60 mg

LOVASTATIN/NIACIN

LOE va sta tin/NYE a sin

TRADE NAME(S):
Advicor

THERAPEUTIC CLASS:
Antilipemic

GENERAL USES:
Hyperlipidemia

DOSAGE FORMS:
Caplets: 20 mg/1 g, 20 mg/750 mg, 20 mg/500 mg

LOXAPINE

LOKS a peen

TRADE NAME(S):
Loxitane, Loxitane C

THERAPEUTIC CLASS:
Antipsychotic

GENERAL USES:
Psychotic disorders

DOSAGE FORMS:
Capsules: 5 mg, 10 mg, 25 mg, 50 mg; Concentrated solution: 25 mg/mL; Injection: 500 mg

MAGNESIUM SULFATE

mag NEE zhum

TRADE NAME(S):
Magnesium sulfate

THERAPEUTIC CLASS:
Electrolyte

GENERAL USES:
Anticonvulsant, replacement

DOSAGE FORMS:
Injection: 10%, 12.5%, 50%

MAPROTILINE

ma PROE ti leen

TRADE NAME(S):
Ludiomil

THERAPEUTIC CLASS:
Antidepressant

GENERAL USES:
Depression

DOSAGE FORMS:
Tablets: 25 mg, 50 mg, 75 mg

MECLIZINE

MEK li zeen

TRADE NAME(S):
Antivert, Antrizine, Vergon

THERAPEUTIC CLASS:
Antiemetic/antivertigo agent

GENERAL USES:
Motion sickness

DOSAGE FORMS:
Tablets: 12.5 mg, 25 mg, 50 mg; Capsules: 25 mg, 30 mg; Chewable tablets: 25 mg

MEDROXYPROGES-TERONE ACETATE

me DROKS ee proe JES te rone

TRADE NAME(S):
Provera, Cycrin, Amen

THERAPEUTIC CLASS:
Hormone (progestin)

GENERAL USES:
Amenorrhea, uterine bleeding

DOSAGE FORMS:
Tablets: 2.5 mg, 5 mg, 10 mg

MEFENAMIC ACID

me fe NAM ik

TRADE NAME(S):
Ponstel

THERAPEUTIC CLASS:
Anti-inflammatory/ analgesic

GENERAL USES:
Menstrual cramping and pain

DOSAGE FORMS:
Capsules: 250 mg

MEFLOQUINE

ME floe kwin

TRADE NAME(S):
Lariam

THERAPEUTIC CLASS:
Antimalarial

GENERAL USES:
Malaria treatment and prevention

DOSAGE FORMS:
Tablets: 250 mg

MEGESTROL ACETATE

me JES trole

TRADE NAME(S):
Megace

THERAPEUTIC CLASS:
Hormone (progestin)

GENERAL USES:
Appetite enhance-ment, breast/

endometrium cancers
(palliative)
DOSAGE FORMS:
Tablets: 20 mg, 40
mg; Suspension: 40
mg/mL

MELOXICAM
mel OKS i kam
TRADE NAME(S):
Mobic
THERAPEUTIC CLASS:
Anti-inflammatory/
analgesic
GENERAL USES:
Osteoarthritis
DOSAGE FORMS:
Tablets: 7.5 mg

MEPERIDINE
me PER i deen
TRADE NAME(S):
Demerol
THERAPEUTIC CLASS:
Analgesic (narcotic)
GENERAL USES:
Pain
DOSAGE FORMS:
Tablets: 50 mg,
100 mg; Syrup:
50 mg/5 mL; Injection:
25 mg, 50 mg, 75 mg,
100 mg

MEQUINOL/TRETINOIN
ME kwi nole/TRET i noyn
TRADE NAME(S):
Solage
THERAPEUTIC CLASS:
Skin agent (topical)
GENERAL USES:
Aging solar skin spots
DOSAGE FORMS:
Solution: 2%/0.01%

MEROPENEM
mer oh PEN em
TRADE NAME(S):
Merrem IV
THERAPEUTIC CLASS:
Anti-infective
GENERAL USES:
Bacterial infections
DOSAGE FORMS:
Injection: 500 mg, 1 g

MESALAMINE
me SAL a meen
TRADE NAME(S):
Asacol, Pentasa
THERAPEUTIC CLASS:
Gastrointestinal agent
GENERAL USES:
Inflammatory bowel
disease
DOSAGE FORMS:
Delayed release
tablets: 400 mg;

Controlled release
capsules: 250 mg

MESORIDAZINE
mez oh RID a zeen
Trade name(s):
Serentil
Therapeutic Class:
Antipsychotic
General Uses:
Psychotic disorders
Dosage Forms:
Tablets: 10 mg, 25
mg, 50 mg, 100 mg;
Concentrated solution:
25 mg/mL; Injection:
25 mg

MESTRANOL/
NORETHINDRONE
MES tra nole/nor eth IN
drone
Trade name(s):
Genora 1/50, Nelova
1/50M, Norethin
1/50M, Norinyl 1+50,
Necon 1/50, Ortho-
Novum 1/50
Therapeutic Class:
Contraceptive
(monophasic)
General Uses:
Contraception
Dosage Forms:
Tablets: 50 mcg/1 mg

METAPROTERENOL
met a proe TER e nol
Trade name(s):
Alupent
Therapeutic Class:
Bronchodilator
General Uses:
Bronchospasm, asthma
Dosage Forms:
Tablets: 10 mg, 20
mg; Syrup: 10 mg/5
mL; Aerosol: 5 mL, 10
mL; Inhalation solu-
tion: 0.4%, 0.6%, 5%

METAXALONE
me TAKS a lone
Trade name(s):
Skelaxin
Therapeutic Class:
Skeletal muscle relax-
ant
General Uses:
Musculoskeletal condi-
tions
Dosage Forms:
Tablets: 400 mg

METFORMIN
met FOR min
Trade name(s):
Glucophage,
Glucophage XR
Therapeutic Class:
Antidiabetic

GENERAL USES:
Diabetes (type 2)
DOSAGE FORMS:
Tablets: 500 mg, 850
mg, 1000 mg;
Extended release
tablets: 500 mg

METHIMAZOLE
meth IM a zole
TRADE NAME(S):
Tapazole
THERAPEUTIC CLASS:
Antithyroid agent
GENERAL USES:
Hyperthyroidism
DOSAGE FORMS:
Tablets: 5 mg, 10 mg

METHOCARBAMOL
meth oh KAR ba mole
TRADE NAME(S):
Robaxin
THERAPEUTIC CLASS:
Skeletal muscle relax-
ant
GENERAL USES:
Musculoskeletal condi-
tions
DOSAGE FORMS:
Tablets: 500 mg, 750
mg

METHOTREXATE
meth oh TREKS ate
TRADE NAME(S):
Rheumatrex
THERAPEUTIC CLASS:
Antineoplastic,
antirheumatic
GENERAL USES:
Cancer, rheumatoid
arthritis
DOSAGE FORMS:
Tablets: 2.5 mg;
Injection: 20 mg, 50
mg, 250 mg, 1 g

METHYLDOPA
meth il DOE pa
TRADE NAME(S):
Aldomet
THERAPEUTIC CLASS:
Antihypertensive
GENERAL USES:
Hypertension
DOSAGE FORMS:
Tablets: 125 mg, 250
mg, 500 mg;
Suspension: 250 mg/5
mL; Injection: 250 mg
(methyldopate)

METHYLDOPA/HCTZ
meth il DOE pa/hye droe
klor oh THYE a zide
TRADE NAME(S):
Aldoril

THERAPEUTIC CLASS:
Antihypertensive/
diuretic
GENERAL USES:
Hypertension
DOSAGE FORMS:
Tablets: 250 mg/15
mg, 250 mg/25 mg,
500 mg/30 mg,
500 mg/50 mg

METHYLPHENIDATE
meth il FEN i date
TRADE NAME(S):
Concerta, Metadate,
Ritalin
THERAPEUTIC CLASS:
CNS stimulant
GENERAL USES:
Attention-deficit disor-
ders, narcolepsy
DOSAGE FORMS:
Tablets: 5 mg, 10 mg,
20 mg; Sustained
release tablets or cap-
sules: 20 mg;
Extended release
tablets: 10 mg, 18 mg,
20 mg, 36 mg, 54 mg

METHYLPRED-
NISOLONE
meth il pred NIS oh lone
TRADE NAME(S):
Medrol

THERAPEUTIC CLASS:
Glucocorticoid
GENERAL USES:
Endocrine, skin, blood
disorders
DOSAGE FORMS:
Tablets: 2 mg, 4 mg,
8 mg, 16 mg, 24 mg,
32 mg

METHYLPRED-
NISOLONE ACETATE
meth il pred NIS oh lone
TRADE NAME(S):
Depo-Medrol,
Depoject, Depopred
THERAPEUTIC CLASS:
Glucocorticoid
GENERAL USES:
Endocrine, skin, blood
disorders
DOSAGE FORMS:
Injection: 40 mg, 80
mg, 100 mg, 200 mg,
400 mg

METHYLPRED-
NISOLONE SODIUM
SUCCINATE
meth il pred NIS oh lone
TRADE NAME(S):
A-Methapred, Solu-
Medrol
THERAPEUTIC CLASS:
Glucocorticoid

GENERAL USES:
Endocrine, skin, blood disorders

DOSAGE FORMS:
Injection: 40 mg, 125 mg, 500 mg, 1 g, 2g

METHYSERGIDE
meth i SER jide

TRADE NAME(S):
Sansert

THERAPEUTIC CLASS:
Antimigraine agent

GENERAL USES:
Migraines

DOSAGE FORMS:
Tablets: 2 mg

METIPRANOLOL
met i PRAN oh lol

TRADE NAME(S):
OptiPranolol

THERAPEUTIC CLASS:
Ocular agent

GENERAL USES:
Glaucoma/ocular hypertension

DOSAGE FORMS:
Ophthalmic solution: 0.3%

METOCLOPRAMIDE
met oh kloe PRA mide

TRADE NAME(S):
Reglan, Clopra, Maxolon, Octamide, Reclomide

THERAPEUTIC CLASS:
Antiemetic

GENERAL USES:
Nausea, vomiting

DOSAGE FORMS:
Tablets: 5 mg, 10 mg; Syrup: 5 mg/5 mL; Concentrated solution: 10 mg/mL; Injection: 10 mg, 50 mg, 150 mg

METOLAZONE
me TOLE a zone

TRADE NAME(S):
Mykrox, Zaroxolyn

THERAPEUTIC CLASS:
Diuretic

GENERAL USES:
CHF related edema, hypertension

DOSAGE FORMS:
Tablets: 0.5 mg, 2.5 mg, 5 mg, 10 mg

METOPROLOL
me toe PROE lole

TRADE NAME(S):
Lopressor, Toprol XL

THERAPEUTIC CLASS:
Antihypertensive, antianginal, cardiac

agent

GENERAL USES:
Hypertension, angina, myocardial infarction

DOSAGE FORMS:
Tablets: 50 mg, 100 mg; Extended release tablets: 25 mg, 50 mg, 100 mg, 200 mg; Injection: 5 mg

METOPROLOL/HCTZ

me toe PROE lole/hye dro klor oh THYE a zide

TRADE NAME(S):
Lopressor HCT

THERAPEUTIC CLASS:
Antihypertensive/diuretic

GENERAL USES:
Hypertension

DOSAGE FORMS:
Tablets: 50 mg/25 mg, 100 mg/25 mg, 100 mg/50 mg

METRONIDAZOLE

me troe NI da zole

TRADE NAME(S):
Flagyl, Flagyl IV

THERAPEUTIC CLASS:
Anti-infective

GENERAL USES:
Bacterial infections, gastric ulcers

DOSAGE FORMS:
Tablets: 250 mg, 500 mg; Extended release tablets: 750 mg; Capsules: 375 mg; Injection: 500 mg

METRONIDAZOLE (TOPICAL)

me troe NI da zole

TRADE NAME(S):
MetroGel, MetroLotion, Noritate

THERAPEUTIC CLASS:
Anti-infective (topical)

GENERAL USES:
Rosacea acne

DOSAGE FORMS:
Gel & Lotion: 0.75%; Cream: 1%

METRONIDAZOLE (VAGINAL)

me troe NI da zole

TRADE NAME(S):
MetroGel Vaginal

THERAPEUTIC CLASS:
Vaginal anti-infective

GENERAL USES:
Vaginal bacterial infections

DOSAGE FORMS:
Gel: 0.75%

MEXILETINE
MEKS i le teen
TRADE NAME(S):
Mexitil
THERAPEUTIC CLASS:
Antiarrhythmic
GENERAL USES:
Arrhythmias, tachycardia
DOSAGE FORMS:
Capsules: 150 mg,
200 mg, 250 mg

MEZLOCILLIN
mezz loe SILL in
TRADE NAME(S):
Mezlin
THERAPEUTIC CLASS:
Anti-infective
GENERAL USES:
Bacterial infections
DOSAGE FORMS:
Injection: 1 g, 2 g, 3 g,
4 g, 20 g

MICONAZOLE
mi KON a zole
TRADE NAME(S):
Monistat-3, Monistat-
Derm
THERAPEUTIC CLASS:
Vaginal antifungal
GENERAL USES:
Vaginal candidiasis

DOSAGE FORMS:
Vaginal suppository: 200
mg; Topical cream: 2%

MIDAZOLAM
MID aye zoe lam
TRADE NAME(S):
Versed
THERAPEUTIC CLASS:
Sedative
GENERAL USES:
Preoperative sedation
DOSAGE FORMS:
Syrup: 2 mg/mL;
Injection: 2 mg, 5 mg,
10 mg, 25 mg, 50 mg

MIFEPRISTONE
mi FE pris tone
TRADE NAME(S):
Mifeprex
THERAPEUTIC CLASS:
Progesterone antago-
nist
GENERAL USES:
Abortifacient
DOSAGE FORMS:
Tablets: 200 mg

MIGLITOL
MIG li tol
TRADE NAME(S):
Glyset

THERAPEUTIC CLASS:
　Antidiabetic
GENERAL USES:
　Diabetes (type 2)
DOSAGE FORMS:
　Tablets: 25 mg, 50
　mg, 100 mg

MINOCYCLINE
mi noe SYE kleen
TRADE NAME(S):
　Dynacin, Vectrin,
　Minocin
THERAPEUTIC CLASS:
　Anti-infective
GENERAL USES:
　Bacterial infections
DOSAGE FORMS:
　Capsules: 50 mg, 100
　mg; Suspension: 50
　mg/5 mL

MINOXIDIL
mi NOKS i dil
TRADE NAME(S):
　Loniten
THERAPEUTIC CLASS:
　Antihypertensive
GENERAL USES:
　Hypertension
DOSAGE FORMS:
　Tablets: 2.5 mg, 10
　mg

MIRTAZAPINE
mir TAZ a peen
TRADE NAME(S):
　Remeron
THERAPEUTIC CLASS:
　Antidepressant
GENERAL USES:
　Depression
DOSAGE FORMS:
　Tablets & Orally disin-
　tegrating tablets: 15
　mg, 30 mg, 45 mg

MISOPROSTOL
mye soe PROST ole
TRADE NAME(S):
　Cytotec
THERAPEUTIC CLASS:
　Gastric protectant
GENERAL USES:
　Prevention of NSAID
　gastric ulcer
DOSAGE FORMS:
　Tablets: 100 mcg, 200
　mcg

MODAFANIL
moe DAF i nil
TRADE NAME(S):
　Provigil
THERAPEUTIC CLASS:
　CNS stimulant
GENERAL USES:
　Narcolepsy

DOSAGE FORMS:
Tablets: 100 mg,
200 mg

MOEXIPRIL/HCTZ
mo EKS i pril/hye droe
klor oh THYE a zide
TRADE NAME(S):
Uniretic
THERAPEUTIC CLASS:
Antihypertensive/
diuretic
GENERAL USES:
Hypertension
DOSAGE FORMS:
Tablets: 15 mg/25 mg,
7.5 mg/12.5 mg

MOLINDONE
moe LIN done
TRADE NAME(S):
Moban
THERAPEUTIC CLASS:
Antipsychotic
GENERAL USES:
Psychotic disorders
DOSAGE FORMS:
Tablets: 5 mg, 10 mg,
25 mg, 50 mg, 100
mg; Concentrated
solution: 20 mg/mL

MOMETASONE
(NASAL)
moe MET a sone
TRADE NAME(S):
Nasonex
THERAPEUTIC CLASS:
Corticosteroid (nasal)
GENERAL USES:
Allergies
DOSAGE FORMS:
Nasal spray: 50
mcg/spray

MOMETASONE
(TOPICAL)
moe MET a sone
TRADE NAME(S):
Elocon
THERAPEUTIC CLASS:
Corticosteroid (topical)
GENERAL USES:
Various skin conditions
DOSAGE FORMS:
Ointment, Cream &
Lotion: 0.1%

MONTELUKAST
mon te LOO kast
TRADE NAME(S):
Singulair
THERAPEUTIC CLASS:
Bronchodilator
GENERAL USES:
Asthma prevention
and treatment

DOSAGE FORMS:
Tablets: 10 mg;
Chewable tablets: 4
mg, 5 mg

MORICIZINE
mor I siz een
TRADE NAME(S):
Ethmozine
THERAPEUTIC CLASS:
Antiarrhythmic
GENERAL USES:
Arrhythmias
DOSAGE FORMS:
Tablets: 200 mg, 250
mg, 300 mg

MORPHINE
MOR feen
TRADE NAME(S):
MS Contin, Oramorph
SR, Kadian, Roxanol,
Duramorph, Infumorph
THERAPEUTIC CLASS:
Analgesic (narcotic)
GENERAL USES:
Pain
DOSAGE FORMS:
Tablets: 15 mg, 30
mg; Controlled release
tablets: 15 mg, 30 mg,
60 mg, 100 mg, 200
mg; Soluble tablets:
10 mg, 15 mg, 30 mg;
Capsules: 15 mg,
30 mg; Sustained
release capsules: 20
mg, 50 mg, 100 mg;
Solution: various con-
centrations; Injection:
various concentrations

MOXIFLOXACIN
moxs i FLOKS a sin
TRADE NAME(S):
Avelox
THERAPEUTIC CLASS:
Anti-infective
GENERAL USES:
Bacterial infections
DOSAGE FORMS:
Tablets: 400 mg;
Injection: 400 mg

MUPIROCIN
myoo PEER oh sin
TRADE NAME(S):
Bactroban
THERAPEUTIC CLASS:
Anti-infective (topical)
GENERAL USES:
Impetigo, skin infec-
tions
DOSAGE FORMS:
Ointment & Cream: 2%

MYCOPHENOLATE MOFETIL

mye koe FEN oh late MOE feh till

TRADE NAME(S):
CellCept

THERAPEUTIC CLASS:
Immunosuppressant

GENERAL USES:
Prevent organ transplant rejection

DOSAGE FORMS:
Capsules: 250 mg; Tablets: 500 mg; Suspension: 200 mg/mL

NABUMETONE

na BYOO me tone

TRADE NAME(S):
Relafen

THERAPEUTIC CLASS:
Anti-inflammatory/ analgesic

GENERAL USES:
Osteoarthritis, rheumatoid arthritis

DOSAGE FORMS:
Tablets: 500 mg, 750 mg

NADOLOL

nay DOE lole

TRADE NAME(S):
Corgard

THERAPEUTIC CLASS:
Antihypertensive, antianginal

GENERAL USES:
Hypertension, angina

DOSAGE FORMS:
Tablets: 20 mg, 40 mg, 80 mg, 120 mg, 160 mg

NAFCILLIN

naf SIL in

TRADE NAME(S):
Unipen, Nallpen

THERAPEUTIC CLASS:
Anti-infective

GENERAL USES:
Bacterial infections

DOSAGE FORMS:
Capsules: 250 mg; Injection: 500 mg, 1 g, 2 g, 10 g

NAFTIFINE

NAF ti feen

TRADE NAME(S):
Naftin

THERAPEUTIC CLASS:
Antifungal (topical)

GENERAL USES:
Athlete's foot, jock itch, ringworm

DOSAGE FORMS:
Cream & Gel: 1%

NALOXONE

nal OKS one

TRADE NAME(S):
Narcan

THERAPEUTIC CLASS:
Antidote

GENERAL USES:
Reversal of opioid effects

DOSAGE FORMS:
Injection: 0.04 mg, 0.4 mg, 0.8 mg, 2 mg, 4 mg, 10 mg

NALTREXONE

nal TREKS one

TRADE NAME(S):
ReVia

THERAPEUTIC CLASS:
Narcotic antagonist

GENERAL USES:
Treatment of alcohol dependence; blocks narcotic effects

DOSAGE FORMS:
Tablets: 50 mg

NAPHAZOLINE

naf AZ oh leen

TRADE NAME(S):
AK-Con, Albalon, Vasocon

THERAPEUTIC CLASS:
Ocular agent

GENERAL USES:
Ocular irritation

DOSAGE FORMS:
Ophthalmic solution: 0.1%

NAPROXEN

na PROKS en

TRADE NAME(S):
Anaprox DS, Aleve, Naprelan

THERAPEUTIC CLASS:
Anti-inflammatory/ analgesic

GENERAL USES:
Osteoarthritis, rheumatoid arthritis, pain

DOSAGE FORMS:
Tablets: 200 mg, 250 mg, 375 mg, 500 mg; Delayed release or Controlled release tablets: 375 mg, 500 mg; Suspension: 125 mg/5 mL

NARATRIPTAN

NAR a trip tan

TRADE NAME(S):
Amerge

THERAPEUTIC CLASS:
Antimigraine agent

GENERAL USES:
Migraines

Dosage Forms:
Tablets: 1 mg, 2.5 mg

NATEGLINIDE
na te GLYE nide
Trade name(s):
Starlix
Therapeutic Class:
Antidiabetic
General Uses:
Diabetes (type 2)
Dosage Forms:
Tablets: 60 mg, 120 mg

NEDOCROMIL
ne doe KROE mil
Trade name(s):
Tilade
Therapeutic Class:
Respiratory inhalant
General Uses:
Asthma
Dosage Forms:
Inhaler: 1.75 mg/inhalation

NEFAZODONE
nef AY zoe done
Trade name(s):
Serzone
Therapeutic Class:
Antidepressant
General Uses:

Depression
Dosage Forms:
Tablets: 50 mg, 100 mg, 150 mg, 200 mg, 250 mg

NELFINAVIR
nel FIN a veer
Trade name(s):
Viracept
Therapeutic Class:
Antiviral
General Uses:
HIV infection
Dosage Forms:
Tablets: 250 mg; Powder: 50 mg/g

NESIRITIDE CITRATE
ni SIR i tide
Trade name(s):
Natrecor
Therapeutic Class:
Cardiac agent
General Uses:
Congestive heart failure
Dosage Forms:
Injection: 1.5 mg

NEVIRAPINE
ne VYE ra peen
Trade name(s):
Viramune

THERAPEUTIC CLASS:
  Antiviral
GENERAL USES:
  HIV infection
DOSAGE FORMS:
  Tablets: 200 mg;
  Suspension: 50 mg/5
  mL

NICARDIPINE
nye KAR de peen
TRADE NAME(S):
  Cardene, Cardene SR,
  Cardene IV
THERAPEUTIC CLASS:
  Antihypertensive,
  antianginal
GENERAL USES:
  Hypertension, angina
DOSAGE FORMS:
  Capsules: 20 mg, 30
  mg; Sustained release
  capsules: 30 mg, 45
  mg, 60 mg; Injection:
  25 mg

NIFEDIPINE
nye FED i peen
TRADE NAME(S):
  Adalat, Procardia,
  Adalat CC, Procardia
  XL
THERAPEUTIC CLASS:
  Antihypertensive (sus-
  tained release),
  antianginal
GENERAL USES:
  Hypertension, angina
DOSAGE FORMS:
  Capsules: 10 mg, 20
  mg; Sustained release
  tablets: 30 mg, 60 mg,
  90 mg

NILUTAMIDE
ni LOO ta mide
TRADE NAME(S):
  Nilandron
THERAPEUTIC CLASS:
  Antiandrogen/antineo-
  plastic
GENERAL USES:
  Prostate cancer
DOSAGE FORMS:
  Tablets: 50 mg

NIMODIPINE
nye MOE di peen
TRADE NAME(S):
  Nimotop
THERAPEUTIC CLASS:
  Cardiac agent
GENERAL USES:
  Brain hemorrhage
DOSAGE FORMS:
  Capsules: 30 mg

NISOLDIPINE
NYE sole di peen

Trade name(s):
Sular
Therapeutic Class:
Antihypertensive
General Uses:
Hypertension
Dosage Forms:
Extended release tablets: 10 mg, 20 mg, 30 mg, 40 mg

NITROGLYCERIN (INJECTION)

nye troe GLI ser in
Trade name(s):
Tridil, Nitro-Bid IV
Therapeutic Class:
Antianginal
General Uses:
Angina
Dosage Forms:
Injection: 5 mg, 25 mg, 50 mg, 100 mg

NITROGLYCERIN (SUBLINGUAL)

nye troe GLI ser in
Trade name(s):
NitroQuick, Nitrostat, Nitrolingual, Nitrotab
Therapeutic Class:
Antianginal
General Uses:
Angina

Dosage Forms:
Sublingual tablets: 0.3 mg, 0.4 mg, 0.6 mg; Spray: 0.4 mg/spray

NITROGLYCERIN (SUSTAINED RELEASE)

nye troe GLI ser in
Trade name(s):
Nitrong, Nitroglyn, Nitro-Time
Therapeutic Class:
Antianginal
General Uses:
Angina
Dosage Forms:
Sustained release tablets: 2.6 mg, 6.5 mg, 9 mg; Sustained release capsules: 2.5 mg, 6.5 mg, 9 mg, 13 mg

NITROGLYCERIN (TOPICAL)

nye troe GLI ser in
Trade name(s):
Nitrol, Nitro-Bid
Therapeutic Class:
Antianginal (topical)
General Uses:
Angina
Dosage Forms:
Ointment: 2%

NITROGLYCERIN (TRANSDERMAL)

nye troe GLI ser in

TRADE NAME(S):
Minitran, Nitro-Dur, Transderm-Nitro, Deponit

THERAPEUTIC CLASS:
Antianginal

GENERAL USES:
Angina

DOSAGE FORMS:
Release rate (mg/hr): 0.1 mg, 0.2 mg, 0.3 mg, 0.4 mg, 0.6 mg, 0.8 mg

NITROGLYCERIN (TRANSMUCOSAL-BUCCAL)

nye troe GLI ser in

TRADE NAME(S):
Nitrogard

THERAPEUTIC CLASS:
Antianginal

GENERAL USES:
Angina

DOSAGE FORMS:
Controlled release tablets: 2 mg, 3 mg

NIZATIDINE

ni ZA ti deen

TRADE NAME(S):
Axid AR, Axid

THERAPEUTIC CLASS:
Antiulcer agent

GENERAL USES:
Duodenal ulcer, GERD, heartburn (OTC)

DOSAGE FORMS:
Tablets: 75 mg; Capsules: 150 mg, 300 mg

NORETHINDRONE

nor eth IN drone

TRADE NAME(S):
Micronor, Nor-QD

THERAPEUTIC CLASS:
Contraceptive (progestin only)

GENERAL USES:
Contraception

DOSAGE FORMS:
Tablets: 0.35 mg

NORETHINDRONE ACETATE

nor eth IN drone

TRADE NAME(S):
Aygestin

THERAPEUTIC CLASS:
Hormone (progestin)

GENERAL USES:
Amenorrhea, endometriosis

DOSAGE FORMS:
Tablets: 5 mg

NORFLOXACIN (OCULAR)
nor FLOKS a sin
Trade name(s):
Chibroxin
Therapeutic Class:
Ocular agent (anti-infective)
General Uses:
Ocular infections
Dosage Forms:
Ophthalmic solution: 3 mg/mL

NORFLOXACIN (ORAL)
nor FLOKS a sin
Trade name(s):
Noroxin
Therapeutic Class:
Anti-infective
General Uses:
Bacterial infections
Dosage Forms:
Tablets: 400 mg

NORGESTREL
nor JES trel
Trade name(s):
Ovrette
Therapeutic Class:
Contraceptive (progestin only)
General Uses:
Contraception

Dosage Forms:
Tablets: 0.075 mg

NORTRIPTYLINE
nor TRIP ti leen
Trade name(s):
Aventyl, Pamelor
Therapeutic Class:
Antidepressant
General Uses:
Depression
Dosage Forms:
Capsules: 10 mg, 25 mg, 50 mg, 75 mg; Solution: 10 mg/5 mL

NYSTATIN (ORAL)
nye STAT in
Trade name(s):
Nilstat, Mycostatin
Therapeutic Class:
Antifungal
General Uses:
Oral fungal infections (candidiasis)
Dosage Forms:
Suspension: 100,000 units/mL; Troches: 200,000 units; Tablets: 500,000 units

NYSTATIN (VAGINAL)
nye STAT in

Therapeutic Class:
Vaginal antifungal
General Uses:
Vaginal candidiasis
Dosage Forms:
Vaginal tablets:
100,000 units

OCTREOTIDE
ok TREE oh tide
Trade name(s):
Sandostatin,
Sandostatin LAR
Depot
Therapeutic Class:
Hormone
General Uses:
Acromegaly, carcinoid
tumors
Dosage Forms:
Injection: 0.05 mg, 0.1
mg, 0.5 mg, 1 mg, 5
mg, 10 mg, 20 mg,
30 mg

OFLOXACIN
oh FLOKS a sin
Trade name(s):
Floxin
Therapeutic Class:
Anti-infective
General Uses:
Bacterial infections

Dosage Forms:
Tablets: 200 mg, 300
mg, 400 mg; Injection:
200 mg, 400 mg

OFLOXACIN
(OCULAR)
oh FLOKS a sin
Trade name(s):
Ocuflox
Therapeutic Class:
Ocular agent (anti-
infective)
General Uses:
Ocular infections
Dosage Forms:
Ophthalmic solution:
3 mg/mL

OLANZAPINE
oh LAN za peen
Trade name(s):
Zyprexa
Therapeutic Class:
Antipsychotic
General Uses:
Psychotic disorders
Dosage Forms:
Tablets: 2.5 mg, 5 mg,
7.5 mg, 10 mg, 15
mg; Orally disintegrat-
ing tablets: 5 mg, 10
mg

OLMESARTAN

ole meh SAR tan

TRADE NAME(S):
Benicar

THERAPEUTIC CLASS:
Antihypertensive

GENERAL USES:
Hypertension

DOSAGE FORMS:
Tablets: 5 mg, 20 mg,
40 mg

OLOPATADINE

oh loe pa TA deen

TRADE NAME(S):
Patanol

THERAPEUTIC CLASS:
Ocular agent

GENERAL USES:
Allergic conjunctivitis

DOSAGE FORMS:
Ophthalmic solution:
0.1%

OLSALAZINE

ol SAL a zeen

TRADE NAME(S):
Dipentum

THERAPEUTIC CLASS:
Gastrointestinal agent

GENERAL USES:
Ulcerative colitis

DOSAGE FORMS:
Capsules: 250 mg

OMEPRAZOLE

oh ME pray zol

TRADE NAME(S):
Prilosec

THERAPEUTIC CLASS:
Gastric acid secretion
inhibitor

GENERAL USES:
Duodenal ulcer, GERD

DOSAGE FORMS:
Delayed release cap-
sules: 10 mg, 20 mg,
40 mg

ONDANSETRON

on DAN se tron

TRADE NAME(S):
Zofran

THERAPEUTIC CLASS:
Antiemetic

GENERAL USES:
Surgical or chemother-
apy nausea/vomiting

DOSAGE FORMS:
Tablets: 4 mg, 8 mg,
24 mg; Solution: 4
mg/5 mL; Orally disin-
tegrating tablets: 4
mg, 8 mg; Injection: 4
mg, 32 mg, 80 mg

ORLISTAT

OR li stat

TRADE NAME(S):
Xenical

THERAPEUTIC CLASS:
Antiobesity
GENERAL USES:
Obesity
DOSAGE FORMS:
Capsules: 120 mg

ORPHENADRINE
or FEN a dreen
TRADE NAME(S):
Norflex
THERAPEUTIC CLASS:
Skeletal muscle relaxant
GENERAL USES:
Musculoskeletal conditions
DOSAGE FORMS:
Tablets & Sustained release tablets: 100 mg

OSELTAMIVIR
oh sel TAM i vir
TRADE NAME(S):
Tamiflu
THERAPEUTIC CLASS:
Anti-influenza
GENERAL USES:
Influenza A or B
DOSAGE FORMS:
Tablets: 75 mg

OXACILLIN
oks a SIL in
TRADE NAME(S):
Oxacillin
THERAPEUTIC CLASS:
Anti-infective
GENERAL USES:
Bacterial infections
DOSAGE FORMS:
Capsules: 250 mg, 500 mg; Solution: 250 mg/5 mL; Injection: 250 mg, 500 mg, 1 g, 2 g, 4 g, 10 g

OXALIPLATIN
ox AL i pla tin
TRADE NAME(S):
Eloxatin
THERAPEUTIC CLASS:
Antineoplastic
GENERAL USES:
Colon or rectal cancer (metastatic)
DOSAGE FORMS:
Injection: 50 mg, 100 mg

OXAPROZIN
oks a PROE zin
TRADE NAME(S):
Daypro
THERAPEUTIC CLASS:
Anti-inflammatory/ analgesic

GENERAL USES:
Osteoarthritis, rheumatoid arthritis
DOSAGE FORMS:
Tablets: 600 mg

OXAZEPAM
oks A ze pam
TRADE NAME(S):
Serax
THERAPEUTIC CLASS:
Antianxiety agent
GENERAL USES:
Anxiety
DOSAGE FORMS:
Tablets: 15 mg; Capsules: 10 mg, 15 mg, 30 mg

OXCARBAZEPINE
ox car BAZ e peen
TRADE NAME(S):
Trileptal
THERAPEUTIC CLASS:
Anticonvulsant
GENERAL USES:
Partial seizures (children)
DOSAGE FORMS:
Tablets: 150 mg, 300 mg, 600 mg; Suspension: 300 mg/5 mL

OXYBUTYNIN
oks i BYOO ti nin
TRADE NAME(S):
Ditropan, Ditropan XL
THERAPEUTIC CLASS:
Antispasmodic
GENERAL USES:
Bladder instability
DOSAGE FORMS:
Tablets: 5 mg; Extended release tablets: 5 mg, 10 mg, 15 mg; Syrup: 5 mg/5 mL

OXYCODONE
oks i KOE done
TRADE NAME(S):
Percolone, Roxicodone, OxyContin, OxyIR, OxyFast
THERAPEUTIC CLASS:
Analgesic (narcotic)
GENERAL USES:
Pain
DOSAGE FORMS:
Tablets: 5 mg; Capsules: 5 mg; Controlled release tablets: 10 mg, 20 mg, 40 mg, 80 mg; Solution: 5 mg/5 mL; Concentrated solution: 20 mg/mL

OXYTOCIN
oks i TOE sin
TRADE NAME(S):
Pitocin, Syntocinon
THERAPEUTIC CLASS:
Oxytocic
GENERAL USES:
Stimulant for labor
DOSAGE FORMS:
Injection: 5 units, 10 units, 100 units

PANCURONIUM
pan kyoo ROE nee um
TRADE NAME(S):
Pavulon
THERAPEUTIC CLASS:
Muscle relaxant
GENERAL USES:
Muscle relaxation for intubation
DOSAGE FORMS:
Injection: 4 mg, 10 mg

PANTOPRAZOLE
pan TOE pra zole
TRADE NAME(S):
Protonix
THERAPEUTIC CLASS:
Gastric acid secretion inhibitor
GENERAL USES:
Erosive esophagitis/ GERD
DOSAGE FORMS:
Delayed release tablets: 40 mg; Injection: 40 mg

PAPAVERINE
pa PAV er een
TRADE NAME(S):
Pavabid, Pavacot
THERAPEUTIC CLASS:
Cardiac agent
GENERAL USES:
Peripheral and cerebral ischemia
DOSAGE FORMS:
Sustained release capsules: 150 mg

PAROMOMYCIN
par oh moe MYE sin
TRADE NAME(S):
Humatin
THERAPEUTIC CLASS:
Antituberculosis agent
GENERAL USES:
Tuberculosis
DOSAGE FORMS:
Capsules: 250 mg

PAROXETINE
pa ROKS e teen
TRADE NAME(S):
Paxil
THERAPEUTIC CLASS:

Antidepressant
GENERAL USES:
Depression, obsessive-compulsive disorder, panic, social anxiety
DOSAGE FORMS:
Tablets: 10 mg, 20 mg, 30 mg, 40 mg; Controlled release tablets: 12.5 mg, 25 mg, 37.5 mg; Suspension: 10 mg/5 mL

PEGINTERFERON ALFA-2b
peg in ter FEER on
TRADE NAME(S):
Peg-Intron
THERAPEUTIC CLASS:
Antiviral
GENERAL USES:
Hepatitis C
DOSAGE FORMS:
Injection: 50 mcg, 80 mcg, 120 mcg, 150 mcg

PEMOLINE
PEM oh leen
TRADE NAME(S):
Cylert
THERAPEUTIC CLASS:
CNS stimulant

GENERAL USES:
Attention-deficit disorders
DOSAGE FORMS:
Tablets: 18.75 mg, 37.5 mg, 75 mg; Chewable tablets: 37.5 mg

PENBUTOLOL
pen BYOO toe lole
TRADE NAME(S):
Levatol
THERAPEUTIC CLASS:
Antihypertensive
GENERAL USES:
Hypertension
DOSAGE FORMS:
Tablets: 20 mg

PENCICLOVIR
pen SYE kloe veer
TRADE NAME(S):
Denavir
THERAPEUTIC CLASS:
Antiviral (topical)
GENERAL USES:
Cold sores, oral herpes
DOSAGE FORMS:
Cream: 1%

PENICILLIN G (AQUEOUS)
pen i SIL in

Trade name(s):
Penicillin G Potassium,
Pfizerpen
Therapeutic Class:
Anti-infective
General Uses:
Bacterial infections
Dosage Forms:
Injection: 1 MU, 2 MU,
3 MU, 5 MU, 10 MU,
20 MU

PENICILLIN G BENZATHINE
pen i SIL in jee BENZ a theen
Trade name(s):
Bicillin LA, Permapen
Therapeutic Class:
Anti-infective
General Uses:
Bacterial infections
Dosage Forms:
Injection: 600,000
units, 1.2 MU, 2.4 MU,
3 MU

PENICILLIN G PROCAINE
pen i SIL in jee PROE kane
Trade name(s):
Wycillin
Therapeutic Class:
Anti-infective

General Uses:
Bacterial infections
Dosage Forms:
Injection: 600,000
units, 1.2 MU, 2.4 MU

PENICILLIN VK
pen i SIL in
Trade name(s):
Beepen-VK, Pen-Vee
K, Veetids
Therapeutic Class:
Anti-infective
General Uses:
Bacterial infections
Dosage Forms:
Tablets: 250 mg, 500
mg; Solution: 125
mg/5 mL,
250 mg/5 mL

PENTAMIDINE ISETHIONATE
pen TAM i deen ice uh THIGH uh nate
Trade name(s):
Pentam 300,
NebuPent
Therapeutic Class:
Anti-infective
General Uses:
Treatment or preven-
tion of pneumonia in
HIV infection

DOSAGE FORMS:
Injection & Aerosol:
300 mg

PENTOBARBITAL
pen toe BAR bi tal
TRADE NAME(S):
Nembutal
THERAPEUTIC CLASS:
Sedative/hypnotic
GENERAL USES:
Insomnia (short term
therapy), pre-op seda-
tive
DOSAGE FORMS:
Capsules: 50 mg, 100
mg; Elixir: 18.2 mg/5
mL; Injection: 1 g, 2.5 g

PENTOXIFYLLINE
pen toks I fi leen
TRADE NAME(S):
Pentoxil, Trental
THERAPEUTIC CLASS:
Blood viscosity reduc-
er agent
GENERAL USES:
Intermittent claudica-
tion
DOSAGE FORMS:
Tablets, Controlled
release tablets,
Extended release
tablets: 400 mg

PERGOLIDE
PER go lide
TRADE NAME(S):
Permax
THERAPEUTIC CLASS:
Antiparkinson agent
GENERAL USES:
Parkinson's disease
DOSAGE FORMS:
Tablets: 0.05 mg, 0.25
mg, 1 mg

PERMETHRIN
per METH rin
TRADE NAME(S):
Elimite, Acticin, Nix
THERAPEUTIC CLASS:
Scabicide/pediculicide
(topical)
GENERAL USES:
Scabies, head lice
DOSAGE FORMS:
Cream: 5%; Crème
rinse: 1%

PERPHENAZINE
per FEN a zeen
TRADE NAME(S):
Trilafon
THERAPEUTIC CLASS:
Antipsychotic
GENERAL USES:
Psychotic disorders
DOSAGE FORMS:
Tablets: 2 mg, 4 mg, 8

mg, 16 mg;
Concentrated solution:
16 mg/5 mL; Injection:
5 mg

PERPHENAZINE/
AMITRIPTYLINE
per FEN a zeen/a mee
TRIP ti leen
TRADE NAME(S):
  Etrafon, Triavil
THERAPEUTIC CLASS:
  Sedative/antidepres-
  sant
GENERAL USES:
  Depression/anxiety
DOSAGE FORMS:
  Tablets: 2 mg/10 mg,
  2 mg/25 mg, 4 mg/25
  mg, 4 mg/50 mg

PHENELZINE
FEN el zeen
TRADE NAME(S):
  Nardil
THERAPEUTIC CLASS:
  Antidepressant
GENERAL USES:
  Depression
DOSAGE FORMS:
  Tablets: 15 mg

PHENOBARBITAL
fee noe BAR bi tal
TRADE NAME(S):
  Barbita, Solfoton
THERAPEUTIC CLASS:
  Sedative/hypnotic,
  anticonvulsant
GENERAL USES:
  Seizures, insomnia
  (short term therapy)
DOSAGE FORMS:
  Tablets: 8 mg, 15 mg,
  16 mg, 30 mg, 60 mg,
  90 mg, 100 mg;
  Capsules: 16 mg;
  Elixir: 15 mg/5 mL, 20
  mg/5 mL; Injection: 60
  mg, 65 mg, 130 mg

PHENTERMINE
FEN ter meen
TRADE NAME(S):
  Fastin, Zantryl, Adipex-
  P, Ionamin
THERAPEUTIC CLASS:
  Anorexiant
GENERAL USES:
  Obesity
DOSAGE FORMS:
  Tablets: 8 mg, 37.5
  mg; Capsules: 15 mg,
  18.75 mg, 30 mg, 37.5
  mg

PHENYTOIN

FEN i toyn

TRADE NAME(S):
Dilantin

THERAPEUTIC CLASS:
Anticonvulsant

GENERAL USES:
Seizures

DOSAGE FORMS:
Chewable tablets: 50 mg; Suspension: 125 mg/5 mL; Extended release tablets: 30 mg, 100 mg; Prompt capsules: 100 mg; Injection: 100 mg, 250 mg

PILOCARPINE (OCULAR)

pye loe KAR peen

TRADE NAME(S):
Isopto Carpine, Pilocar, Akarpine, Pilostat

THERAPEUTIC CLASS:
Ocular agent

GENERAL USES:
Glaucoma

DOSAGE FORMS:
Ophthalmic solution: 0.25%, 0.5%, 1%, 2%, 3%, 4%, 5%, 6%, 8%, 10%; Ophthalmic gel: 4%

PILOCARPINE (ORAL)

pye loe KAR peen

TRADE NAME(S):
Salagen

THERAPEUTIC CLASS:
Saliva stimulant

GENERAL USES:
Saliva deficiency

DOSAGE FORMS:
Tablets: 5 mg

PIMECROLIMUS

pim eh KROE lih muss

TRADE NAME(S):
Elidel

THERAPEUTIC CLASS:
Anti-inflammatory agent

GENERAL USES:
Ezcema

DOSAGE FORMS:
Cream: 1%

PIMOZIDE

PI moe zide

TRADE NAME(S):
Orap

THERAPEUTIC CLASS:
Antipsychotic

GENERAL USES:
Tourette's

DOSAGE FORMS:
Tablets: 2 mg

PINDOLOL
PIN doe lole
TRADE NAME(S):
Visken
THERAPEUTIC CLASS:
Antihypertensive
GENERAL USES:
Hypertension
DOSAGE FORMS:
Tablets: 5 mg, 10 mg

PIOGLITAZONE
pye oh GLI ta zone
TRADE NAME(S):
Actos
THERAPEUTIC CLASS:
Antidiabetic
GENERAL USES:
Diabetes (type 2)
DOSAGE FORMS:
Tablets: 15 mg, 30 mg, 45 mg

PIPERACILLIN
pi PER a sil in
TRADE NAME(S):
Pipracil
THERAPEUTIC CLASS:
Anti-infective
GENERAL USES:
Bacterial infections
DOSAGE FORMS:
Injection: 2 g, 3 g, 4 g, 40 g

PIPERACILLIN/ TAZOBACTAM
pi PER a sil in/ta zoe BAK tam
TRADE NAME(S):
Zosyn
THERAPEUTIC CLASS:
Anti-infective
GENERAL USES:
Bacterial infections
DOSAGE FORMS:
Injection: 2 g/0.25 g, 3 g/0.375 g, 4 g/0.5 g, 36 g/4.5 g

PIRBUTEROL
peer BYOO ter ole
TRADE NAME(S):
Maxair
THERAPEUTIC CLASS:
Bronchodilator
GENERAL USES:
Bronchospasm, asthma
DOSAGE FORMS:
Inhaler: 0.2 mg/inhalation

PIROXICAM
peer OKS i kam
TRADE NAME(S):
Feldene
THERAPEUTIC CLASS:
Anti-inflammatory/ analgesic
GENERAL USES:

Osteoarthritis, rheuma-
toid arthritis

DOSAGE FORMS:
Capsules: 10 mg,
20 mg

POTASSIUM CHLORIDE

poe TASS ee um KLOR
ide

TRADE NAME(S):
K-Dur, Kaon-Cl, Klor-
Con, Klotrix, Klorvess,
K-Lyte, Micro-K

THERAPEUTIC CLASS:
Electrolyte (potassium)

GENERAL USES:
Potassium replace-
ment

DOSAGE FORMS:
Controlled release or
Extended release
tablets: 6.7 mEq, 8
mEq, 10 mEq;
Effervescent tablets:
20 mEq, 25 mEq, 50
mEq; Liquid: 20 mEq,
30 mEq or 40 mEq/15
mL; Powder: 20 mEq,
25 mEq; Injection: var-
ious concentrations

PRAMIPEXOLE

pra mi PEKS ole

TRADE NAME(S):
Mirapex

THERAPEUTIC CLASS:
Antiparkinson agent

GENERAL USES:
Parkinson's disease

DOSAGE FORMS:
Tablets: 0.125 mg,
0.25 mg, 0.5 mg, 1
mg, 1.5 mg

PRAVASTATIN

PRA va stat in

TRADE NAME(S):
Pravachol

THERAPEUTIC CLASS:
Antilipemic

GENERAL USES:
Hyperlipidemia

DOSAGE FORMS:
Tablets: 10 mg, 20
mg, 40 mg

PRAZOSIN

PRA zoe sin

TRADE NAME(S):
Minipress

THERAPEUTIC CLASS:
Antihypertensive

GENERAL USES:
Hypertension

DOSAGE FORMS:
Capsules: 1 mg, 2 mg,
5 mg

PRAZOSIN/ POLYTHIAZIDE

PRA zoe sin/pol i THYE a zide

TRADE NAME(S):
Minizide

THERAPEUTIC CLASS:
Antihypertensive/diuretic

GENERAL USES:
Hypertension

DOSAGE FORMS:
Capsules: 1 mg/0.5 mg, 2 mg/0.5 mg, 5 mg/0.5 mg

PREDNISOLONE (OCULAR)

pred NISS oh lone

TRADE NAME(S):
Pred Mild, Econopred, Pred Forte

THERAPEUTIC CLASS:
Ocular agent (steroid)

GENERAL USES:
Ocular inflammation

DOSAGE FORMS:
Ophthalmic suspension & Solution: 0.1%, 0.125%

PREDNISOLONE (ORAL)

pred NISS oh lone

TRADE NAME(S):
Prelone, Delta-Cortef

THERAPEUTIC CLASS:
Glucocorticoid

GENERAL USES:
Endocrine, skin, blood disorders

DOSAGE FORMS:
Tablets: 5 mg; Syrup: 5 mg/5 mL, 15 mg/5 mL

PREDNISONE

PRED ni sone

TRADE NAME(S):
Deltasone, Prednicen-M, Meticorten, Panasol-S

THERAPEUTIC CLASS:
Glucocorticoid

GENERAL USES:
Endocrine, skin, blood disorders

DOSAGE FORMS:
Tablets: 1 mg, 2.5 mg, 5 mg, 10 mg, 20 mg, 50 mg; Syrup & Solution: 5 mg/5 mL; Concentrated solution: 5 mg/mL

PRIMAQUINE

PRIM a kween

TRADE NAME(S):
Primaquine

THERAPEUTIC CLASS:

Antimalarial
GENERAL USES:
Malaria treatment
DOSAGE FORMS:
Tablets: 26.3 mg

PRIMIDONE
PRI mi done
TRADE NAME(S):
Mysoline
THERAPEUTIC CLASS:
Anticonvulsant
GENERAL USES:
Seizures
DOSAGE FORMS:
Tablets: 50 mg, 250 mg; Suspension: 250 mg/5 mL

PROBENECID
proe BEN e sid
TRADE NAME(S):
Benemid, Probalan
THERAPEUTIC CLASS:
Gout agent
GENERAL USES:
Gout
DOSAGE FORMS:
Tablets: 500 mg

PROCAINAMIDE
proe kane A mide
TRADE NAME(S):
Pronestyl, Procanbid

THERAPEUTIC CLASS:
Antiarrhythmic
GENERAL USES:
Arrhythmias
DOSAGE FORMS:
Tablets: 250 mg, 375 mg, 500 mg; Sustained release tablets: 250 mg, 500 mg, 750 mg, 1000 mg; Capsules: 250 mg, 375 mg, 500 mg; Injection: 1 g

PROCHLORPERAZINE
proe klor PER a zeen
TRADE NAME(S):
Compazine
THERAPEUTIC CLASS:
Antiemetic, antipsychotic
GENERAL USES:
Emesis, psychotic disorders, anxiety
DOSAGE FORMS:
Tablets: 5 mg, 10 mg, 25 mg; Sustained release capsules: 10 mg, 15 mg, 30 mg; Syrup: 5 mg/5 mL; Injection: 10 mg, 50 mg

PROCYCLIDINE
proe SYE kli deen

TRADE NAME(S):
Kemadrin
THERAPEUTIC CLASS:
Antiparkinson agent
GENERAL USES:
Parkinson's disease, drug induced extrapyramidal disorders
DOSAGE FORMS:
Tablets: 5 mg

PROGESTERONE
proe JES ter one
TRADE NAME(S):
Prometrium
THERAPEUTIC CLASS:
Hormone (progesterone)
GENERAL USES:
Amenorrhea, uterine bleeding
DOSAGE FORMS:
Capsules: 100 mg; Vaginal gel: 4%, 8%

PROPAFENONE
proe pa FEEN one
TRADE NAME(S):
Rythmol
THERAPEUTIC CLASS:
Antiarrhythmic
GENERAL USES:
Arrhythmias, tachycardia

DOSAGE FORMS:
Tablets: 150 mg, 225 mg, 300 mg

PROPANTHELINE
proe PAN the leen
TRADE NAME(S):
Pro-Banthine
THERAPEUTIC CLASS:
Gastrointestinal agent
GENERAL USES:
Peptic ulcer
DOSAGE FORMS:
Tablets: 7.5 mg, 15 mg

PROPOXYPHENE
proe POKS i feen
TRADE NAME(S):
Darvon-N, Darvon
THERAPEUTIC CLASS:
Analgesic (narcotic)
GENERAL USES:
Pain
DOSAGE FORMS:
Tablets: 100 mg; Capsules: 65 mg

PROPRANOLOL
proe PRAN oh lole
TRADE NAME(S):
Inderal, Inderal LA, Betachron ER
THERAPEUTIC CLASS:

Cardiac agent, antimigraine

GENERAL USES:
Hypertension, angina, MI, migraines, essential tremor

DOSAGE FORMS:
Tablets: 10 mg, 20 mg, 40 mg, 60 mg, 80 mg, 90 mg; Sustained release & Extended release capsules: 60 mg, 80 mg, 120 mg, 160 mg; Solution: 4 mg/mL, 8 mg/mL; Concentrated solution: 80 mg/mL; Injection: 1 mg

PROPRANOLOL/HCTZ
proe PRAN oh lole/hye droe klor oh THYE a zide

TRADE NAME(S):
Inderide, Inderide LA

THERAPEUTIC CLASS:
Antihypertensive/ diuretic

GENERAL USES:
Hypertension

DOSAGE FORMS:
Tablets: 40 mg/25 mg, 80 mg/25 mg; Long acting capsules: 80 mg/50 mg, 120 mg/50 mg, 160 mg/50 mg

PROPYLTHIOURACIL
proe pil thye oh YOOR a sil

TRADE NAME(S):
Propylthiouracil

THERAPEUTIC CLASS:
Antithyroid agent

GENERAL USES:
Hyperthyroidism

DOSAGE FORMS:
Tablets: 50 mg

PROTRIPTYLINE
proe TRIP ti leen

TRADE NAME(S):
Vivactil

THERAPEUTIC CLASS:
Antidepressant

GENERAL USES:
Depression

DOSAGE FORMS:
Tablets: 5 mg, 10 mg

PYRAZINAMIDE
peer a ZIN a mide

TRADE NAME(S):
Pyrazinamide

THERAPEUTIC CLASS:
Antituberculosis agent

GENERAL USES:
Tuberculosis

DOSAGE FORMS:
Tablets: 500 mg

QUAZEPAM
KWAY ze pam
TRADE NAME(S):
Doral
THERAPEUTIC CLASS:
Sedative/hypnotic
GENERAL USES:
Insomnia
DOSAGE FORMS:
Tablets: 7.5 mg, 15 mg

QUETIAPINE
kwe TYE a peen
TRADE NAME(S):
Seroquel
THERAPEUTIC CLASS:
Antipsychotic
GENERAL USES:
Psychotic disorders
DOSAGE FORMS:
Tablets: 25 mg, 100 mg, 200 mg, 300 mg

QUINAPRIL
KWIN a pril
TRADE NAME(S):
Accupril
THERAPEUTIC CLASS:
Antihypertensive, cardiac agent
GENERAL USES:
Hypertension, heart failure
DOSAGE FORMS:
Tablets: 5 mg, 10 mg, 20 mg, 40 mg

QUINIDINE GLUCONATE
KWIN i deen
TRADE NAME(S):
Quinaglute, Quinalan
THERAPEUTIC CLASS:
Antiarrhythmic
GENERAL USES:
Atrial fibrillation, tachycardia
DOSAGE FORMS:
Sustained release tablets: 324 mg; Injection: 800 mg

QUINIDINE SULFATE
KWIN i deen
TRADE NAME(S):
Quinora, Quinidex Extentabs
THERAPEUTIC CLASS:
Antiarrhythmic
GENERAL USES:
Atrial fibrillation, tachycardia
DOSAGE FORMS:
Tablets: 200 mg, 300 mg; Extended release tablets: 300 mg

QUININE SULFATE
KWYE nine
TRADE NAME(S):
Quinine
THERAPEUTIC CLASS:
Antimalarial
GENERAL USES:
Chloroquine resistant malaria
DOSAGE FORMS:
Capsules: 200 mg, 260 mg, 325 mg; Tablets: 260 mg

RABEPRAZOLE
ra BE pray zole
TRADE NAME(S):
Aciphex
THERAPEUTIC CLASS:
Gastric acid secretion inhibitor
GENERAL USES:
GERD, duodenal ulcer, hyperacidity disorders
DOSAGE FORMS:
Delayed release tablets: 20 mg

RALOXIFENE
ral OKS i feen
TRADE NAME(S):
Evista
THERAPEUTIC CLASS:
Hormones (estrogen modulator)
GENERAL USES:
Osteoporosis prevention
DOSAGE FORMS:
Tablets: 60 mg

RAMIPRIL
ra MI pril
TRADE NAME(S):
Altace
THERAPEUTIC CLASS:
Antihypertensive, cardiac agent
GENERAL USES:
Hypertension, CHF
DOSAGE FORMS:
Capsules: 1.25 mg, 2.5 mg, 5 mg, 10 mg

RANITIDINE
ra NI ti deen
TRADE NAME(S):
Zantac 75, Zantac EFFERdose, Zantac GELdose
THERAPEUTIC CLASS:
Gastric acid secretion inhibitor
GENERAL USES:
Duodenal ulcer, GERD, heartburn (OTC)
DOSAGE FORMS:
Tablets: 75 mg; Tablets and Capsules: 150 mg, 300 mg;

Effervescent tablets/granules: 150 mg; Syrup: 15 mg/mL; Injection: 50 mg, 150 mg, 1 g

RASBURICASE
ras BYOOR i kayse
TRADE NAME(S):
 Elitek
THERAPEUTIC CLASS:
 Antigout
GENERAL USES:
 Gout related to chemotherapy/cancer
DOSAGE FORMS:
 Injection: 1.5 mg

REPAGLINIDE
re pa GLI nide
TRADE NAME(S):
 Prandin
THERAPEUTIC CLASS:
 Antidiabetic
GENERAL USES:
 Diabetes (type 2)
DOSAGE FORMS:
 Tablets: 0.5 mg, 1 mg, 2 mg

RETEPLASE
RE ta plase
TRADE NAME(S):
 Retavase
THERAPEUTIC CLASS:
 Thrombolytic agent
GENERAL USES:
 Dissolves blood clots in MI
DOSAGE FORMS:
 Injection: 10.8 IU (18.8 mg)

RIBAVIRIN (AEROSOL)
rye ba VYE rin
TRADE NAME(S):
 Virazole
THERAPEUTIC CLASS:
 Antiviral
GENERAL USES:
 Severe lower respiratory tract infections in infants
DOSAGE FORMS:
 Aerosol: 6 g

RIBAVIRIN (ORAL)
rye ba VYE rin
TRADE NAME(S):
 Rebetrol
THERAPEUTIC CLASS:
 Antiviral
GENERAL USES:
 Chronic hepatitis C
DOSAGE FORMS:
 Capsules: 200 mg

RIFABUTIN
rif a BYOO tin
TRADE NAME(S):
Mycobutin
THERAPEUTIC CLASS:
Antituberculosis agent
GENERAL USES:
Tuberculosis
DOSAGE FORMS:
Capsules: 150 mg

RIFAMPIN
RIF am pin
TRADE NAME(S):
Rifadin, Rimactane
THERAPEUTIC CLASS:
Antituberculosis agent
GENERAL USES:
Tuberculosis
DOSAGE FORMS:
Capsules: 150 mg,
300 mg; Injection:
600 mg

RIFAPENTINE
RIF a pen teen
TRADE NAME(S):
Priftin
THERAPEUTIC CLASS:
Antituberculosis agent
GENERAL USES:
Tuberculosis
DOSAGE FORMS:
Tablets: 150 mg

RILUZOLE
RIL yoo zole
TRADE NAME(S):
Rilutek
THERAPEUTIC CLASS:
Amyotrophic lateral
sclerosis agent
GENERAL USES:
Amyotrophic lateral
sclerosis
DOSAGE FORMS:
Tablets: 50 mg

RIMANTADINE
ri MAN ta deen
TRADE NAME(S):
Flumadine
THERAPEUTIC CLASS:
Antiviral
GENERAL USES:
Influenza A
DOSAGE FORMS:
Tablets: 100 mg;
Syrup: 50 mg/5 mL

RIMEXOLONE
ri MEKS oh lone
TRADE NAME(S):
Vexol
THERAPEUTIC CLASS:
Ocular agent
GENERAL USES:
Postoperative ocular
inflammation

DOSAGE FORMS:
Ophthalmic suspension: 1%

RISEDRONATE
ris ED roe nate
TRADE NAME(S):
Actonel
THERAPEUTIC CLASS:
Bisphosphonate
GENERAL USES:
Paget's disease, osteoporosis
DOSAGE FORMS:
Tablets: 5 mg, 30 mg

RISPERIDONE
ris PER i done
TRADE NAME(S):
Risperdal
THERAPEUTIC CLASS:
Antipsychotic
GENERAL USES:
Psychotic disorders
DOSAGE FORMS:
Tablets: 0.25 mg, 0.5 mg,1 mg, 2 mg, 3 mg, 4 mg; Solution: 1 mg/mL

RITONAVIR
ri TOE na veer
TRADE NAME(S):
Norvir
THERAPEUTIC CLASS:
Antiviral
GENERAL USES:
HIV infection
DOSAGE FORMS:
Capsules: 100 mg; Solution: 80 mg/mL

RIVASTIGMINE
ri va STIG meen
TRADE NAME(S):
Exelon
THERAPEUTIC CLASS:
Alzheimer's agent
GENERAL USES:
Alzheimer's disease
DOSAGE FORMS:
Capsules: 1.5 mg, 3 mg, 4.5 mg, 6 mg; Solution: 2 mg/mL

RIZATRIPTAN
rye za TRIP tan
TRADE NAME(S):
Maxalt, Maxalt-MLT
THERAPEUTIC CLASS:
Antimigraine agent
GENERAL USES:
Migraines
DOSAGE FORMS:
Tablets & orally disintegrating tablets: 5 mg, 10 mg

ROFECOXIB
roe fe COX ib
TRADE NAME(S):
Vioxx
THERAPEUTIC CLASS:
Anti-inflammatory/
analgesic
GENERAL USES:
Osteoarthritis, acute
pain, menstrual pain
DOSAGE FORMS:
Tablets: 12.5 mg, 25
mg; Suspension: 12.5
mg/5 mL, 25 mg/5 mL

ROPINIROLE
roe PIN i role
TRADE NAME(S):
Requip
THERAPEUTIC CLASS:
Antiparkinson agent
GENERAL USES:
Parkinson's disease
DOSAGE FORMS:
Tablets: 0.25 mg, 0.5
mg, 1 mg, 2 mg, 5 mg

ROSIGLITAZONE
roh si GLI ta zone
TRADE NAME(S):
Avandia
THERAPEUTIC CLASS:
Antidiabetic
GENERAL USES:
Diabetes (type 2)

DOSAGE FORMS:
Tablets: 2 mg, 4 mg,
8 mg

SACROSIDASE
sak ROE si dase
TRADE NAME(S):
Sucraid
THERAPEUTIC CLASS:
Enzyme replacement
GENERAL USES:
Sucrase-isomaltase
deficiency
DOSAGE FORMS:
Solution: 8500 IU/mL

SALSALATE
SAL sa late
TRADE NAME(S):
Disalcid, Amigesic;
Salsitab
THERAPEUTIC CLASS:
Anti-inflammatory/
analgesic
GENERAL USES:
Pain, osteoarthritis,
rheumatoid arthritis
DOSAGE FORMS:
Capsules: 500 mg;
Tablets: 500 mg, 750 mg

SAQUINAVIR
sa KWIN a veer

TRADE NAME(S):
Invirase, Fortovase
THERAPEUTIC CLASS:
Antiviral
GENERAL USES:
HIV infection
DOSAGE FORMS:
Capsules: 200 mg

SCOPOLAMINE
skoe POL a meen
TRADE NAME(S):
Transderm-Scop
THERAPEUTIC CLASS:
Antiemetic/antivertigo
agent
GENERAL USES:
Motion sickness
DOSAGE FORMS:
Transdermal patch:
1.5 mg

SECOBARBITAL
see koe BAR bi tal
TRADE NAME(S):
Seconal
THERAPEUTIC CLASS:
Sedative/hypnotic
GENERAL USES:
Insomnia (short term
therapy)
DOSAGE FORMS:
Capsules: 100 mg

SELEGILINE
se LE ji leen
TRADE NAME(S):
Eldepryl, Carbex
THERAPEUTIC CLASS:
Antiparkinson agent
GENERAL USES:
Parkinson's disease
DOSAGE FORMS:
Tablets: 5 mg;
Capsules: 5 mg

SERTRALINE
SER tra leen
TRADE NAME(S):
Zoloft
THERAPEUTIC CLASS:
Antidepressant
GENERAL USES:
Depression, obsessive
compulsive disorder,
panic disorder
DOSAGE FORMS:
Tablets: 25 mg, 50 mg,
100 mg; Concentrated
solution: 20 mg/mL

SIBUTRAMINE
si BYOO tra meen
TRADE NAME(S):
Meridia
THERAPEUTIC CLASS:
Anorexiant
GENERAL USES:
Obesity

DOSAGE FORMS:
Capsules: 5 mg, 10 mg, 15 mg

SILDENAFIL
sil DEN a fil
TRADE NAME(S):
Viagra
THERAPEUTIC CLASS:
Impotence agent
GENERAL USES:
Erectile dysfunction
DOSAGE FORMS:
Tablets: 25 mg, 50 mg, 100 mg

SIMVASTATIN
SIM va stat in
TRADE NAME(S):
Zocor
THERAPEUTIC CLASS:
Antilipemic
GENERAL USES:
Hyperlipidemia, coronary heart disease
DOSAGE FORMS:
Tablets: 5 mg, 10 mg, 20 mg, 40 mg, 80 mg

SIROLIMUS
sir OH li mus
TRADE NAME(S):
Rapamune
THERAPEUTIC CLASS:

Immunomodulator
GENERAL USES:
Prevent organ transplant rejection
DOSAGE FORMS:
Solution: 1 mg/mL; Tablets: 1 mg

SOTALOL
SOE ta lole
TRADE NAME(S):
Betapace, Betapace AF
THERAPEUTIC CLASS:
Antiarrhythmic
GENERAL USES:
Arrhythmias
DOSAGE FORMS:
Tablets: 80 mg, 120 mg, 160 mg, 240 mg

SPARFLOXACIN
spar FLOKS a sin
TRADE NAME(S):
Zagam
THERAPEUTIC CLASS:
Anti-infective
GENERAL USES:
Bacterial infections
DOSAGE FORMS:
Tablets: 200 mg

SPIRONOLACTONE
speer on oh LAK tone
TRADE NAME(S):
  Aldactone
THERAPEUTIC CLASS:
  Diuretic
GENERAL USES:
  Edema, hypertension,
  hyperaldosteronism
DOSAGE FORMS:
  Tablets: 25 mg, 50
  mg, 100 mg

STAVUDINE (d4T)
STAV yoo deen
TRADE NAME(S):
  Zerit
THERAPEUTIC CLASS:
  Antiviral
GENERAL USES:
  HIV infection
DOSAGE FORMS:
  Capsules: 15 mg, 20
  mg, 30 mg, 40 mg;
  Powder: 1 mg/mL

STREPTOKINASE
strep toe KYE nase
TRADE NAME(S):
  Streptase
THERAPEUTIC CLASS:
  Thrombolytic agent
GENERAL USES:
  Dissolves blood clots

DOSAGE FORMS:
  Injection: 250,000 IU,
  750,000 IU, 1.5 million
  IU

SUCRALFATE
soo KRAL fate
TRADE NAME(S):
  Carafate
THERAPEUTIC CLASS:
  Gastric protectant
GENERAL USES:
  Duodenal ulcer
DOSAGE FORMS:
  Tablets: 1 g;
  Suspension: 1 g/10
  mL

SULFADIAZINE
sul fa DYE a zeen
TRADE NAME(S):
  Microsulfon
THERAPEUTIC CLASS:
  Anti-infective
GENERAL USES:
  Bacterial infections
DOSAGE FORMS:
  Tablets: 500 mg

SULFASALAZINE
sul fa SAL a zeen
TRADE NAME(S):
  Azulfidine, Azulfidine
  EN

THERAPEUTIC CLASS:
Gastrointestinal agent
GENERAL USES:
Ulcerative colitis,
rheumatoid arthritis
DOSAGE FORMS:
Tablets: 500 mg;
Delayed release
tablets: 500 mg

SULFINPYRAZONE
sul fin PEER a zone
TRADE NAME(S):
Anturane
THERAPEUTIC CLASS:
Gout agent
GENERAL USES:
Gouty arthritis
DOSAGE FORMS:
Tablets: 100 mg;
Capsules: 200 mg

SULINDAC
sul IN dak
TRADE NAME(S):
Clinoril
THERAPEUTIC CLASS:
Anti-inflammatory/
analgesic
GENERAL USES:
Various arthritis condi-
tions, pain
DOSAGE FORMS:
Tablets: 150 mg,
200 mg

SUMATRIPTAN
soo ma TRIP tan
TRADE NAME(S):
Imitrex
THERAPEUTIC CLASS:
Antimigraine
GENERAL USES:
Migraine
DOSAGE FORMS:
Tablets: 25 mg, 50
mg, 100 mg; Nasal
spray: 5 mg, 20 mg;
Injection: 6 mg

SUPROFEN
soo PRO fen
TRADE NAME(S):
Profenal
THERAPEUTIC CLASS:
Ocular agent
GENERAL USES:
Maintain pupil dilation
during surgery
DOSAGE FORMS:
Ophthalmic solution: 1%

TACRINE
TAK reen
TRADE NAME(S):
Cognex
THERAPEUTIC CLASS:
Alzheimer's agent
GENERAL USES:
Alzheimer's disease

DOSAGE FORMS:
 Capsules: 10 mg, 20 mg, 30 mg, 40 mg

TACROLIMUS
ta KROE li mus
TRADE NAME(S):
 Prograf
THERAPEUTIC CLASS:
 Immunosuppressant
GENERAL USES:
 Prevent organ transplant rejection
DOSAGE FORMS:
 Capsules: 1 mg, 5 mg

TAMOXIFEN
ta MOKS i fen
TRADE NAME(S):
 Nolvadex
THERAPEUTIC CLASS:
 Antiestrogen/antineoplastic
GENERAL USES:
 Breast cancer
DOSAGE FORMS:
 Tablets: 10 mg, 20 mg

TAMSULOSIN
tam SOO loe sin
TRADE NAME(S):
 Flomax
THERAPEUTIC CLASS:
 Urologic agent

GENERAL USES:
 Benign prostatic hypertrophy
DOSAGE FORMS:
 Capsules: 0.4 mg

TAZAROTENE
taz AR oh teen
TRADE NAME(S):
 Tazorac
THERAPEUTIC CLASS:
 Retinoid (topical)
GENERAL USES:
 Acne, psoriasis
DOSAGE FORMS:
 Gel: 0.05%, 0.1%

TEGASEROD
teg a SER od
TRADE NAME(S):
 Zelnorm
THERAPEUTIC CLASS:
 Gastrointestinal agent
GENERAL USES:
 Irritable bowel syndrome (women)
DOSAGE FORMS:
 Tablets: 2 mg, 6 mg

TELMISARTAN
tel mi SAR tan
TRADE NAME(S):
 Micardis
THERAPEUTIC CLASS:

Antihypertensive
GENERAL USES:
Hypertension
DOSAGE FORMS:
Tablets: 40 mg, 80 mg

TEMAZEPAM
te MAZ e pam
TRADE NAME(S):
Restoril
THERAPEUTIC CLASS:
Sedative/hypnotic
GENERAL USES:
Insomnia
DOSAGE FORMS:
Capsules: 7.5 mg, 15 mg, 30 mg

TEMOZOLOMIDE
te moe ZOE loe mide
TRADE NAME(S):
Temodar
THERAPEUTIC CLASS:
Antineoplastic
GENERAL USES:
Astrocytoma (brain tumor)
DOSAGE FORMS:
Capsules: 5 mg, 20 mg, 100 mg, 250 mg

TENECTEPLASE
ten EK te plase
TRADE NAME(S):
TNKase
THERAPEUTIC CLASS:
Thrombolytic
GENERAL USES:
Dissolves blood clots in MI
DOSAGE FORMS:
Injection: 50 mg

TENOFOVIR
te NOE fo veer
TRADE NAME(S):
Viread
THERAPEUTIC CLASS:
Antiviral
GENERAL USES:
HIV infection
DOSAGE FORMS:
Tablets: 300 mg

TERAZOSIN
ter AY zoe sin
TRADE NAME(S):
Hytrin
THERAPEUTIC CLASS:
Antihypertensive, BPH agent
GENERAL USES:
Hypertension, benign prostatic hypertrophy
DOSAGE FORMS:
Capsules, Tablets: 1 mg, 2 mg, 5 mg, 10 mg

TERBINAFINE

TER bin a feen

TRADE NAME(S):
Lamisil

THERAPEUTIC CLASS:
Antifungal

GENERAL USES:
Nail fungal infections, ringworm, athlete's foot

DOSAGE FORMS:
Tablets: 250 mg; Cream & Gel: 1%

TERBUTALINE

ter BYOO ta leen

TRADE NAME(S):
Brethine

THERAPEUTIC CLASS:
Bronchodilator

GENERAL USES:
Bronchospasm, asthma

DOSAGE FORMS:
Tablets: 2.5 mg, 5 mg; Inhaler: 0.2 mg/inhalation; Injection: 1 mg

TERCONAZOLE

ter KONE a zole

TRADE NAME(S):
Terazol-7, Terazol-3

THERAPEUTIC CLASS:
Vaginal antifungal

GENERAL USES:
Vaginal candidiasis

DOSAGE FORMS:
Vaginal cream: 0.4%, 0.8%; Vaginal suppository: 80 mg

TESTOSTERONE (TOPICAL)

tes TOS ter one

TRADE NAME(S):
Androgel

THERAPEUTIC CLASS:
Hormone

GENERAL USES:
Replacement therapy in men

DOSAGE FORMS:
Gel: 1%

TESTOSTERONE (TRANSDERMAL)

tes TOS ter one

TRADE NAME(S):
Androderm

THERAPEUTIC CLASS:
Hormone

GENERAL USES:
Replacement therapy in men

DOSAGE FORMS:
Patch: 2.5 mg/24 hrs, 5 mg/24 hrs

TETRACYCLINE
tet ra SYE kleen
TRADE NAME(S):
  Sumycin, Tetracyn
THERAPEUTIC CLASS:
  Anti-infective
GENERAL USES:
  Bacterial infections
DOSAGE FORMS:
  Capsules & Tablets:
  250 mg, 500 mg;
  Suspension: 125 mg/5
  mL

THALIDOMIDE
tha LI doe mide
TRADE NAME(S):
  Thalomid
THERAPEUTIC CLASS:
  Immunomodulator
GENERAL USES:
  Erythema nodosum
  leprosum (skin disor-
  der)
DOSAGE FORMS:
  Capsules: 50 mg

THEOPHYLLINE
thee OFF i lin
TRADE NAME(S):
  Slo-Phyllin, Theo-Dur,
  several others
THERAPEUTIC CLASS:
  Bronchodilator

GENERAL USES:
  Bronchial asthma,
  bronchospasm
DOSAGE FORMS:
  Tablets: 100 mg, 125
  mg, 200 mg, 250 mg,
  300 mg; Capsules:
  100 mg, 200 mg;
  Syrup & Elixir: 26.7
  mg/5 mL; Syrup: 50
  mg/5 mL; Timed
  release tablets & cap-
  sules: 50 mg, 75 mg,
  100 mg, 125 mg, 200
  mg, 250 mg, 300 mg,
  400 mg, 500 mg, 600
  mg

THIOPENTAL
thye oh PEN tal
TRADE NAME(S):
  Pentothal
THERAPEUTIC CLASS:
  Anesthetic
GENERAL USES:
  Anesthesia
DOSAGE FORMS:
  Injection: 250 mg, 400
  mg, 500 mg, 1 g, 2.5
  g, 5 g

THIORIDAZINE
thye oh RID a zeen
TRADE NAME(S):
  Mellaril, Mellaril-S

THERAPEUTIC CLASS:
Antipsychotic
GENERAL USES:
Psychotic disorders,
emesis
DOSAGE FORMS:
Tablets: 10 mg, 15
mg, 25 mg, 50 mg,
100 mg, 150 mg, 200
mg; Concentrated
solution: 30 mg/mL,
100 mg/mL;
Suspension: 25 mg/5
mL, 100 mg/5 mL

THIOTHIXENE
thye oh THIKS een
TRADE NAME(S):
Navane
THERAPEUTIC CLASS:
Antipsychotic
GENERAL USES:
Psychotic/behavioral
disorders
DOSAGE FORMS:
Capsules: 1 mg, 2 mg,
5 mg, 10 mg,
20 mg; Concentrated
solution: 5 mg/mL

TIAGABINE
tye AG a been
TRADE NAME(S):
Gabitril
THERAPEUTIC CLASS:

Anticonvulsant
GENERAL USES:
Seizures
DOSAGE FORMS:
Tablets: 4 mg, 12 mg,
16 mg, 20 mg

TICARCILLIN
tye kar SIL in
TRADE NAME(S):
Ticar
THERAPEUTIC CLASS:
Anti-infective
GENERAL USES:
Bacterial infections
DOSAGE FORMS:
Injection: 1 g, 3 g, 6 g,
20 g, 30 g

TICARCILLIN/CLAVU-LANATE POTASSIUM
tye kar SIL in/klav yoo
LAN ate
TRADE NAME(S):
Timentin
THERAPEUTIC CLASS:
Anti-infective
GENERAL USES:
Bacterial infections
DOSAGE FORMS:
Injection: 3 g/0.1 g

TICLOPIDINE
tye KLOE pi deen

TRADE NAME(S):
  Ticlid
THERAPEUTIC CLASS:
  Antiplatelet agent
GENERAL USES:
  Reduce risk of stroke
  due to clots
DOSAGE FORMS:
  Tablets: 250 mg

TILUDRONATE
tye LOO droe nate
TRADE NAME(S):
  Skelid
THERAPEUTIC CLASS:
  Bisphosphonate
GENERAL USES:
  Paget's disease
DOSAGE FORMS:
  Tablets: 240 mg

TIMOLOL (OCULAR)
TYE moe lole
TRADE NAME(S):
  Betimol, Timoptic
THERAPEUTIC CLASS:
  Ocular agent
GENERAL USES:
  Glaucoma/ocular
  hypertension
DOSAGE FORMS:
  Ophthalmic solution:
  0.25%, 0.5%

TIMOLOL (ORAL)
TYE moe lole
TRADE NAME(S):
  Blocadren
THERAPEUTIC CLASS:
  Antihypertensive, car-
  diac agent, anti-
  migraine agent
GENERAL USES:
  Hypertension, myocar-
  dial infarction,
  migraines
DOSAGE FORMS:
  Tablets: 5 mg, 10 mg,
  20 mg

TIMOLOL/HCTZ
TYE moe lole/hye droe
klor oh THYE a zide
TRADE NAME(S):
  Timolide
THERAPEUTIC CLASS:
  Antihypertensive/
  diuretic
GENERAL USES:
  Hypertension
DOSAGE FORMS:
  Tablets: 10 mg/25 mg

TINZAPARIN
tin ZA pa rin
TRADE NAME(S):
  Innohep
THERAPEUTIC CLASS:
  Anticoagulant (LMWH)

GENERAL USES:
Treatment for deep
vein thrombosis
DOSAGE FORMS:
Injection: 40,000 IU

TIZANIDINE
tye ZAN i deen
TRADE NAME(S):
Zanaflex
THERAPEUTIC CLASS:
Skeletal muscle relax-
ant
GENERAL USES:
Muscle spasticity
DOSAGE FORMS:
Tablets: 4 mg

TOBRAMYCIN
(OCULAR)
toe bra MYE sin
TRADE NAME(S):
Tobrex, AKTob
THERAPEUTIC CLASS:
Ocular agent (anti-
infective)
GENERAL USES:
Ocular infections
DOSAGE FORMS:
Ophthalmic solution:
0.3%; Ophthalmic
ointment: 3 mg/g

TOBRAMYCIN
SULFATE
toe bra MYE sin
TRADE NAME(S):
Nebcin
THERAPEUTIC CLASS:
Anti-infective
GENERAL USES:
Bacterial infections
DOSAGE FORMS:
Injection: 20 mg, 60
mg, 80 mg, 1.2 g;
Nebulizer solution: 300
mg

TOCAINIDE
toe KAY nide
TRADE NAME(S):
Tonocard
THERAPEUTIC CLASS:
Antiarrhythmic
GENERAL USES:
Ventricular arrhythmias
DOSAGE FORMS:
Tablets: 400 mg,
600 mg

TOLAZAMIDE
tole AZ a mide
TRADE NAME(S):
Tolinase
THERAPEUTIC CLASS:
Antidiabetic
GENERAL USES:
Diabetes (type 2)

DOSAGE FORMS:
Tablets: 100 mg, 250 mg, 500 mg

TOLBUTAMIDE
tole BYOO ta mide
TRADE NAME(S):
Orinase
THERAPEUTIC CLASS:
Antidiabetic
GENERAL USES:
Diabetes (type 2)
DOSAGE FORMS:
Tablets: 500 mg

TOLCAPONE
TOLE ka pone
TRADE NAME(S):
Tasmar
THERAPEUTIC CLASS:
Antiparkinson agent
GENERAL USES:
Parkinson's disease
DOSAGE FORMS:
Tablets: 100 mg, 200 mg

TOLMETIN
TOLE met in
TRADE NAME(S):
Tolectin
THERAPEUTIC CLASS:
Anti-inflammatory/ analgesic

GENERAL USES:
Osteoarthritis, rheumatoid arthritis
DOSAGE FORMS:
Tablets: 200 mg, 600 mg; Capsules: 400 mg

TOLTERODINE
tole TER oh deen
TRADE NAME(S):
Detrol, Detrol LA
THERAPEUTIC CLASS:
Antispasmodic
GENERAL USES:
Bladder instability
DOSAGE FORMS:
Tablets: 1 mg, 2 mg; Extended release capsules: 2 mg, 4 mg

TOPIRAMATE
toe PYRE a mate
TRADE NAME(S):
Topamax
THERAPEUTIC CLASS:
Anticonvulsant
GENERAL USES:
Seizures
DOSAGE FORMS:
Tablets: 25 mg, 100 mg, 200 mg; Sprinkle capsules: 15 mg, 25 mg

TOREMIFENE
TORE em i feen
TRADE NAME(S):
Fareston
THERAPEUTIC CLASS:
Antiestrogen/antineo-
plastic
GENERAL USES:
Breast cancer
DOSAGE FORMS:
Tablets: 60 mg

TORSEMIDE
TORE se mide
TRADE NAME(S):
Demadex
THERAPEUTIC CLASS:
Diuretic
GENERAL USES:
CHF related edema,
hypertension
DOSAGE FORMS:
Tablets: 5 mg, 10 mg,
20 mg, 100 mg

TRAMADOL
TRA ma dole
TRADE NAME(S):
Ultram
THERAPEUTIC CLASS:
Analgesic
GENERAL USES:
Pain
DOSAGE FORMS:
Tablets: 50 mg

TRAMADOL/ ACETAMINOPHEN
TRA ma dole/a seet a
MIN oh fen
TRADE NAME(S):
Ultracet
THERAPEUTIC CLASS:
Analgesic
GENERAL USES:
Short term treatment
of pain
DOSAGE FORMS:
Tablets: 37.5 mg/325
mg

TRANDOLAPRIL
tran DOE la pril
TRADE NAME(S):
Mavik
THERAPEUTIC CLASS:
Antihypertensive, car-
diac agent
GENERAL USES:
Hypertension, conges-
tive heart failure
DOSAGE FORMS:
Tablets: 1 mg, 2 mg, 4
mg

TRANDOLAPRIL/ VERAPAMIL
tran DOE la pril/ver AP a
mil
TRADE NAME(S):
Tarka

THERAPEUTIC CLASS:
  Antihypertensive/
  diuretic
GENERAL USES:
  Hypertension
DOSAGE FORMS:
  Tablets: 1 mg/240 mg,
  2 mg/240 mg,
  4 mg/240 mg

TRANYLCYPROMINE
tran il SIP roe meen
TRADE NAME(S):
  Parnate
THERAPEUTIC CLASS:
  Antidepressant
GENERAL USES:
  Depression
DOSAGE FORMS:
  Tablets: 10 mg

TRAVOPROST
TRA voe prost
TRADE NAME(S):
  Travatan
THERAPEUTIC CLASS:
  Ocular agent
GENERAL USES:
  Open angle glaucoma,
  ocular hypertension
DOSAGE FORMS:
  Ophthalmic solution:
  0.004%

TRAZODONE
TRAZ oh done
TRADE NAME(S):
  Desyrel
THERAPEUTIC CLASS:
  Antidepressant
GENERAL USES:
  Depression
DOSAGE FORMS:
  Tablets: 50 mg, 100
  mg, 150 mg, 300 mg

TREPROSTINIL SODIUM
treh PROS tih nill
TRADE NAME(S):
  Remodulin
THERAPEUTIC CLASS:
  Cardiac agent
GENERAL USES:
  Pulmonary arterial
  hypertension
DOSAGE FORMS:
  Injection: 1 mg, 2.5
  mg, 5 mg, 10 mg

TRETINOIN (TOPICAL)
TRET i noyn
TRADE NAME(S):
  Retin-A, Retin-A Micro
THERAPEUTIC CLASS:
  Retinoid (topical)
GENERAL USES:
  Acne vulgaris

DOSAGE FORMS:
Cream & Gel: 0.025%,
0.1%; Cream: 0.05%;
Liquid: 0.05%; Gel:
0.01%

TRIAMCINOLONE (INHALED)
trye am SIN oh lone
TRADE NAME(S):
Azmacort
THERAPEUTIC CLASS:
Corticosteroid (inhaler)
GENERAL USES:
Asthma (chronic)
DOSAGE FORMS:
Inhaler: 100
mcg/inhalation

TRIAMCINOLONE (NASAL)
trye am SIN oh lone
TRADE NAME(S):
Nasacort, Nasacort
AQ
THERAPEUTIC CLASS:
Corticosteroid (nasal)
GENERAL USES:
Allergies
DOSAGE FORMS:
Nasal spray & Inhaler:
55 mcg/spray

TRIAMCINOLONE (ORAL)
trye am SIN oh lone
TRADE NAME(S):
Kenacort, Aristocort
THERAPEUTIC CLASS:
Glucocorticoid
GENERAL USES:
Endocrine, skin, blood
disorders
DOSAGE FORMS:
Tablets: 4 mg, 8 mg;
Syrup: 4 mg/5 mL

TRIAMCINOLONE ACETONIDE
try am SIN oh lone
TRADE NAME(S):
Aristocort, Kenalog,
Flutex
THERAPEUTIC CLASS:
Corticosteroid (topical)
GENERAL USES:
Various skin conditions
DOSAGE FORMS:
Ointment & Cream:
0.025%, 0.1%, 0.5%;
Lotion: 0.025%, 0.1%

TRIAMTERENE
trye AM ter een
TRADE NAME(S):
Dyrenium
THERAPEUTIC CLASS:
Diuretic

GENERAL USES:
CHF related edema, hypertension

DOSAGE FORMS:
Tablets: 50 mg, 100 mg

TRIAZOLAM
trye AY zoe lam

TRADE NAME(S):
Halcion

THERAPEUTIC CLASS:
Sedative/hypnotic

GENERAL USES:
Insomnia

DOSAGE FORMS:
Tablets: 0.125 mg, 0.25 mg

TRIFLUOPERAZINE
trye floo oh PER a zeen

TRADE NAME(S):
Stelazine

THERAPEUTIC CLASS:
Antipsychotic

GENERAL USES:
Psychotic disorders, anxiety

DOSAGE FORMS:
Tablets: 1 mg, 2 mg, 5 mg, 10 mg; Concentrated solution: 10 mg/mL; Injection: 20 mg

TRIFLURIDINE
trye FLURE i deen

TRADE NAME(S):
Viroptic

THERAPEUTIC CLASS:
Ocular agent (antiviral)

GENERAL USES:
Ocular herpes infections

DOSAGE FORMS:
Ophthalmic solution: 1%

TRIHEXYPHENIDYL
trye heks ee FEN i dil

TRADE NAME(S):
Artane

THERAPEUTIC CLASS:
Antiparkinson agent

GENERAL USES:
Parkinson's disease, drug induced extrapyramidal disorders

DOSAGE FORMS:
Tablets: 2 mg, 5 mg; Sustained release capsules: 5 mg; Elixir: 2 mg/5 mL

TRIMETHOPRIM/ SULFAMETHOXAZOLE
trye METH oh prim/sul fa meth OKS a zole

TRADE NAME(S):

Bactrim, Cotrim,
Septra
THERAPEUTIC CLASS:
Anti-infective
GENERAL USES:
Bacterial infections
DOSAGE FORMS:
Tablets: 80 mg/400
mg, 160 mg/800 mg;
Suspension: 40
mg/200 mg/5 mL;
Injection: 800 mg/l60
mg, 1600 mg/320 mg

TRIMIPRAMINE
trye MI pra meen
TRADE NAME(S):
Surmontil
THERAPEUTIC CLASS:
Antidepressant
GENERAL USES:
Depression
DOSAGE FORMS:
Capsules: 25 mg, 50
mg, 100 mg

TRIPTORELIN
PAMOATE
trip toe REL in
TRADE NAME(S):
Trelstar Depot, Trelstar
LA
THERAPEUTIC CLASS:
Antineoplastic
GENERAL USES:

Palliative treatment of
advanced prostate
cancer
DOSAGE FORMS:
Injection: 3.75 mg,
11.25 mg

TROLEANDOMYCIN
troe lee an doe MYE sin
TRADE NAME(S):
TAO
THERAPEUTIC CLASS:
Anti-infective
GENERAL USES:
Bacterial infections
DOSAGE FORMS:
Capsules: 250 mg

UNOPROSTONE
ISOPROPYL
yoo noe PROS tone
TRADE NAME(S):
Rescula
THERAPEUTIC CLASS:
Ocular agent
GENERAL USES:
Open angle glaucoma
DOSAGE FORMS:
Ophthalmic solution:
0.15%

URSODIOL
ER soe dye ole
TRADE NAME(S):

Actigall, Urso
THERAPEUTIC CLASS:
Gallstone solubilizer
GENERAL USES:
Gallstones
DOSAGE FORMS:
Capsules: 300 mg

VALACYCLOVIR
val ay SYE kloe veer
TRADE NAME(S):
Valtrex
THERAPEUTIC CLASS:
Antiviral
GENERAL USES:
Herpes, shingles
DOSAGE FORMS:
Tablets: 500 mg,
1000 mg

VALDECOXIB
val de KOKS ib
TRADE NAME(S):
Bextra
THERAPEUTIC CLASS:
Anti-inflammatory/analgesic
GENERAL USES:
Rheumatoid arthritis,
osteoarthritis, primary
dysmenorrhea
DOSAGE FORMS:
Tablets: 10 mg, 20 mg

VALGANCICLOVIR
val gan SYE kloh veer
TRADE NAME(S):
Valcyte
THERAPEUTIC CLASS:
Antiviral
GENERAL USES:
CMV retinitis in HIV
patients
DOSAGE FORMS:
Tablets: 450 mg

VALPROIC ACID & DERIVATIVES
val PROE ik AS id
TRADE NAME(S):
Depakote, Depakene
THERAPEUTIC CLASS:
Anticonvulsant
GENERAL USES:
Seizures
DOSAGE FORMS:
Capsules: 250 mg;
Delayed release
tablets: 125 mg, 250
mg, 500 mg; Sprinkle
capsules: 125 mg;
Syrup: 250 mg/5 mL;
Injection: 500 mg

VALSARTAN
val SAR tan
TRADE NAME(S):
Diovan
THERAPEUTIC CLASS:

Antihypertensive

GENERAL USES:
Hypertension

DOSAGE FORMS:
Capsules: 80 mg, 160 mg, 320 mg

VALSARTAN/HCTZ
val SAR tan/hye droe klor oh THYE a zide

TRADE NAME(S):
Diovan HCT

THERAPEUTIC CLASS:
Antihypertensive/ diuretic

GENERAL USES:
Hypertension

DOSAGE FORMS:
Tablets: 80 mg/12.5 mg, 160 mg/12.5 mg

VANCOMYCIN
van koe MYE sin

TRADE NAME(S):
Vancocin, Vancoled

THERAPEUTIC CLASS:
Anti-infective

GENERAL USES:
Bacterial infections

DOSAGE FORMS:
Capsules: 125 mg, 250 mg; Solution: 1 g, 10 g; Injection: 500 mg, 1 g, 2 g, 5 g, 10 g

VECURONIUM
ve KYOO roe ni um

TRADE NAME(S):
Norcuron

THERAPEUTIC CLASS:
Muscle relaxant

GENERAL USES:
Aid to anesthesia

DOSAGE FORMS:
Injection: 10 mg, 20 mg

VENLAFAXINE
VEN la faks een

TRADE NAME(S):
Effexor, Effexor XR

THERAPEUTIC CLASS:
Antidepressant

GENERAL USES:
Depression

DOSAGE FORMS:
Tablets: 25 mg, 37.5 mg, 50 mg, 75 mg, 100 mg; Extended release tablets: 37.5 mg, 75 mg, 150 mg

VERAPAMIL
ver AP a mil

TRADE NAME(S):
Calan, Isoptin, Verelan, Isoptin SR, Calan SR, Verelan PM

THERAPEUTIC CLASS:
Antihypertensive (SR),

antianginal
GENERAL USES:
Hypertension, angina
DOSAGE FORMS:
Tablets: 40 mg, 80 mg, 120 mg; Sustained release Tablets & Capsules: 120 mg, 180 mg, 240 mg; Sustained release capsules: 100 mg, 200 mg, 300 mg; Injection: 5 mg

VIDARABINE
vye DARE a been
TRADE NAME(S):
Vira-A
THERAPEUTIC CLASS:
Ocular agent (antiviral)
GENERAL USES:
Ocular herpes infections
DOSAGE FORMS:
Ophthalmic ointment: 3%

VINBLASTINE
vin BLAS teen
TRADE NAME(S):
Velban
THERAPEUTIC CLASS:
Antineoplastic
GENERAL USES:
Various cancers

DOSAGE FOR
Injection:
25 mg

VINCRISTINE
vin KRIS teen
TRADE NAME(S):
Vincasar PFS
THERAPEUTIC CLASS:
Antineoplastic
GENERAL USES:
Various cancers
DOSAGE FORMS:
Injection: 1 mg, 2 mg, 5 mg

VINORELBINE
vi NOR el been
TRADE NAME(S):
Navelbine
THERAPEUTIC CLASS:
Antineoplastic
GENERAL USES:
Various cancers
DOSAGE FORMS:
Injection: 10 mg, 50 mg

VITAMIN K (PHYTONADIONE)
fye toe na DYE one
TRADE NAME(S):
Aqua-Mephyton, Mephyton

...tic Class:
...min

General Uses:
Blood clotting disorders

Dosage Forms:
Tablets: 5 mg;
Injection: 1 mg

VORICONAZOLE
vore ih KON uh zole

Trade name(s):
VFEND

Therapeutic Class:
Antifungal

General Uses:
Serious fungal infections

Dosage Forms:
Tablets: 50 mg, 200 mg; Injection: 200 mg

WARFARIN
WAR far in

Trade name(s):
Coumadin

Therapeutic Class:
Anticoagulant

General Uses:
Preventive therapy for blood clots

Dosage Forms:
Tablets: 1 mg, 2 mg, 2.5 mg, 3 mg, 4 mg, 5 mg, 6 mg, 7.5 mg,
10 mg

ZAFIRLUKAST
za FIR loo kast

Trade name(s):
Accolate

Therapeutic Class:
Bronchodilator

General Uses:
Asthma prevention and treatment

Dosage Forms:
Tablets: 10 mg, 20 mg

ZALCITABINE (ddC)
zal SITE a been

Trade name(s):
Hivid

Therapeutic Class:
Antiviral

General Uses:
HIV infection

Dosage Forms:
Tablets: 0.375 mg, 0.75 mg

ZALEPLON
ZAL e plon

Trade name(s):
Sonata

Therapeutic Class:
Hypnotic/sedative

General Uses:
Insomnia

DOSAGE FORMS:
Capsules: 5 mg, 10 mg

ZANAMIVIR
za NA mi veer
TRADE NAME(S):
Relenza
THERAPEUTIC CLASS:
Antiviral
GENERAL USES:
Influenza A and B
DOSAGE FORMS:
Inhalation: 5
mg/inhalation

ZIDOVUDINE
zye DOE vyoo deen
TRADE NAME(S):
Retrovir
THERAPEUTIC CLASS:
Antiviral
GENERAL USES:
HIV infection
DOSAGE FORMS:
Capsules: 100 mg;
Tablets: 300 mg;
Syrup: 50 mg/mL;
Injection: 200 mg

ZILEUTON
zye LOO ton
TRADE NAME(S):
Zyflo
THERAPEUTIC CLASS:

Antiasthmatic
GENERAL USES:
Asthma prevention
and treatment
DOSAGE FORMS:
Tablets: 600 mg

ZIPRASIDONE
zi PRAY si done
TRADE NAME(S):
Geodon
THERAPEUTIC CLASS:
Antipsychotic
GENERAL USES:
Schizophrenia
DOSAGE FORMS:
Capsules: 20 mg, 40
mg, 60 mg, 80 mg;
Injection: 20 mg

ZOLEDRONIC ACID
ZOE le dron ik AS id
TRADE NAME(S):
Zometa
THERAPEUTIC CLASS:
Bisphosphonate
GENERAL USES:
Treatment of hypercal-
cemia of cancer
DOSAGE FORMS:
Injection: 4 mg

ZOLMITRIPTAN
zohl mi TRIP tan

TRADE NAME(S):
Zomig, Zomig-ZMT

THERAPEUTIC CLASS:
Antimigraine

GENERAL USES:
Migraine

DOSAGE FORMS:
Tablets: 2.5 mg, 5 mg;
Orally disintegrating
tablets: 2.5 mg

ZOLPIDEM
zole PI dem

TRADE NAME(S):
Ambien

THERAPEUTIC CLASS:
Sedative, hypnotic

GENERAL USES:
Insomnia

DOSAGE FORMS:
Tablets: 5 mg, 10 mg

ZONISAMIDE
zoe NIS a mide

TRADE NAME(S):
Zonegran

THERAPEUTIC CLASS:
Anticonvulsant

GENERAL USES:
Partial seizures (adults)

DOSAGE FORMS:
Capsules: 100 mg

Augmentin (amoxicillin/clavu-
lanate), 7

Augmentin ES
(amoxicillin/clavulanate), 7

Avandia (rosiglitazone), 133

Avapro (irbesartan), 82

Avelox (moxifloxacin), 104

Aventyl (nortriptyline), 111

Avonex (interferon beta-1a),
81

Axert (almotriptan), 4

Axid (nizatidine), 110

Axid AR (nizatidine), 110

Aygestin (norethindrone
acetate), 110

Azactam (aztreonam), 12

Azmacort (triamcinolone,
inhaled), 148

Azopt (brinzolamide), 18

Azulfidine (sulfasalazine), 136

Azulfidine EN (sulfasalazine),
136

B

Bactrim (trimethoprim/sul-
famethoxazole), 149

Bactroban (mupirocin), 104

Barbita (phenobarbital), 120

Beclovent (beclomethasone,
inhaled), 13

Beconase (beclomethasone,
nasal), 14

Beconase AQ (beclometha-
sone, nasal), 14

Beepen-VK (penicillin VK), 118

Benadryl (diphenhydramine),
44

Benemid (probenecid), 125

Benicar (olmesartan), 113

Bentyl (dicyclomine), 42

Benzac (benzoyl peroxide),
14

Benzamycin
(erythromycin/benzoyl peroxide), 53

Betachron ER (propranolol),
126

Betagan (levobunolol), 88

Betapace (sotalol), 135

Betapace AF (sotalol), 135

Betaseron (interferon beta-
1b), 82

Betatrex (betamethasone
valerate), 15

Betaxon (levobetaxolol), 88

Betimol (timolol, ocular), 143

Betoptic (betaxolol, ocular),
15

Betoptic S (betaxolol, ocular),
15

Bextra (valdecoxib), 151

Biaxin (clarithromycin), 32

Bicillin LA (penicillin G benza-
thine), 118

Biocef (cephalexin), 27

Blocadren (timolol, oral), 143

Botox (botulinum toxin type
A), 17

Brethine (terbutaline), 140

Brevicon (ethinyl
estradiol/norethindrone), 58

Bronkosol (isoetharine), 83

Bumex (bumetanide), 19

BuSpar (buspirone), 20

Demadex (torsemide), 146

Demerol (meperidine), 95

Demulen 1/35 (ethinyl estra-
diol/ethynodiol), 56

Demulen 1/50 (ethinyl estra-
diol/ethynodiol), 56

Denavir (penciclovir), 117

Depakene (valproic acid &
derivatives), 151

Depakote (valproic acid &
derivatives), 151

Depoject (methylprednisolone
acetate), 98

Depo-Medrol (methylpred-
nisolone acetate), 98

Deponit (nitroglycerin, transdermal), 110

Depopred (methylpred-
nisolone acetate), 98

Dermacort (hydrocortisone,
topical), 76

Desogen (ethinyl
estradiol/desogestrel), 55

DesOwen (desonide), 39

Desyrel (trazodone), 147

Detrol (tolterodine), 145

Detrol LA (tolterodine), 145

Dexasone (dexamethasone
sodium phosphate), 40

Dexedrine (dextroampheta-
mine sulfate), 41

Dexone (dexamethasone,
oral), 40

Diabeta (glyburide), 72

Diabinese (chlorpropamide),
30

Didronel (etidronate), 61

Differin (adapalene), 2

Diflucan (fluconazole), 65

Diflucan IV (fluconazole), 65

Dilacor XR (diltiazem), 44

Dilantin (phenytoin), 121

Diovan (valsartan), 151

Diovan HCT
(valsartan/HCTZ), 152

Dipentum (olsalazine), 113

Diprosone (betamethasone
diproprionate), 15

Disalcid (salsalate), 133

Di-Spaz (dicyclomine), 42

Ditropan (oxybutynin), 115

Ditropan XL (oxybutynin), 115

Diuril (chlorothiazide), 30

Dobutrex (dobutamine), 46

Dolobid (diflunisal), 43

Doral (quazepam), 128

Dostinex (cabergoline), 20

Dovonex (calcipotriene), 20

Doxy (doxycycline), 48

Doxychel (doxycycline), 48

Dramanate (dimenhydrinate),
44

Drithocreme (anthralin), 9

Duragesic (fentanyl, transdermal), 64

Duramorph (morphine), 104

Duricef (cefadroxil), 23

Dycill (dicloxacillin), 42

Dymelor (acetohexamide), 2

Dynabac (dirithromycin), 45

Dynacin (minocycline), 102

DynaCirc (isradipine), 84

DynaCirc CR (isradipine), 84

Dynapen (dicloxacillin), 42

Maxidex (dexamethasone, ocular), 40
Maxipime (cefepime), 24
Maxivate (betamethasone diproprionate), 15
Maxolon (metoclopramide), 99
Medihaler (isoproterenol), 83
Medrol (methylprednisolone), 98
Mefoxin (cefoxitin sodium), 25
Megace (megestrol acetate), 94
Mellaril (thioridazine), 141
Mellaril-S (thioridazine), 141
Menest (estrogens, esterified), 54
Mentax (butenafine), 20
Mephyton (vitamin K [phytonadione]), 153
Meridia (sibutramine), 134
Merrem IV (meropenem), 95
Metadate (methylphenidate), 98
Meticorten (prednisone), 124
MetroGel (metronidazole, topical), 100
MetroGel Vaginal (metronidazole, vaginal), 100
MetroLotion (metronidazole, topical), 100
Mevacor (lovastatin), 93
Mexitil (mexiletine), 101
Mezlin (mezlocillin), 101
Micardis (telmisartan), 138
Micro-K (potassium chloride), 123

Micronase (glyburide), 72
Micronor (norethindrone),110
Microsulfon (sulfadiazine), 136
Midamor (amiloride), 5
Mifeprex (mifepristone),101
Migranal (dihydroergotamine), 43
Minipress (prazosin), 123
Minitran (nitroglycerin, transdermal), 110
Minizide (prazosin/polythiazide), 124
Minocin (minocycline), 102
Mirapex (pramipexole), 123
Mircette (ethinyl estradiol/desogestrel), 55
Mitran (chlordiazepoxide), 29
Moban (molindone), 103
Mobic (meloxicam), 95
Modicon (ethinyl estradiol/norethindrone), 58
Monistat-Derm (miconazole), 101
Monistat-3 (miconazole), 101
Monocid (cefonicid), 25
Monoket (isosorbide mononitrate), 84
Monopril (fosinopril), 69
Motrin (ibuprofen), 77
MS Contin (morphine), 104
Myambutol (ethambutol), 55
Mycelex (clotrimazole, oral), 35
Mycelex (clotrimazole, topical), 35
Mycobutin (rifabutin), 131

T

Tagamet (cimetidine), 31
Tagamet HB (cimetidine), 31
Tambocor (flecainide), 64
Tamiflu (oseltamivir), 114
TAO (troleandomycin), 150
Tapazole (methimazole), 97
Targretin (bexarotene), 16
Tarka (trandolapril/verapamil), 146
Tasmar (tolcapone), 145
Tazidime (ceftazidime), 26
Tazorac (tazarotene), 138
Teczem (diltiazem/enalapril), 44
Tegison (etretinate), 62
Tegretol (carbamazepine), 22
Temodar (temozolomide), 139
Temovate (clobetasol), 33
Tempra (acetaminophen), 1
Tenex (guanfacine), 74
Tenoretic (atenolol/chlorthalidone), 11
Tenormin (atenolol), 11
Tequin (gatifloxacin), 71
Terazol-3 (terconazole), 140
Terazol-7 (terconazole), 140
Tessalon Perles (benzonatate), 14
Tetracyn (tetracycline), 141
Thalitone (chlorthalidone), 30
Thalomid (thalidomide), 141
Theo-Dur (theophylline), 141
Thorazine (chlorpromazine), 30
Tiazac (diltiazem), 44

Ticar (ticarcillin), 142
Ticlid (ticlopidine), 142
Tikosyn (dofetilide), 46
Tilade (nedocromil), 107
Timentin (ticarcillin/clavulanate potassium), 142
Timolide (timolol/HCTZ), 143
Timoptic (timolol, ocular), 143
TNKase (tenecteplase), 139
Tobrex (tobramycin, ocular), 144
Tofranil (imipramine HCl), 78
Tofranil-PM (imipramine pamoate), 79
Tolectin (tolmetin), 145
Tolinase (tolazamide), 144
Tonocard (tocainide), 144
Topamax (topiramate), 145
Toprol XL (metoprolol), 99
Toradol (ketorolac), 85
Tornalate (bitolterol), 17
Totacillin (ampicillin), 8
Tracleer (bosentan), 17
Trandate (labetalol), 86
Transderm-Nitro (nitroglycerin, transdermal), 110
Transderm-Scop (scopolamine), 134
Tranxene (clorazepate), 34
Travatan (travoprost), 147
Trecator-SC (ethionamide), 61
Trelstar Depot (triptorelin pamoate), 150
Trelstar LA (triptorelin pamoate), 150
Trental (pentoxifylline), 119